Marta Tarallo

by hand

Homemade Beauty

A modern guide to making soaps, shampoo bars & skincare essentials

Photography by Luke Albert

quadrille

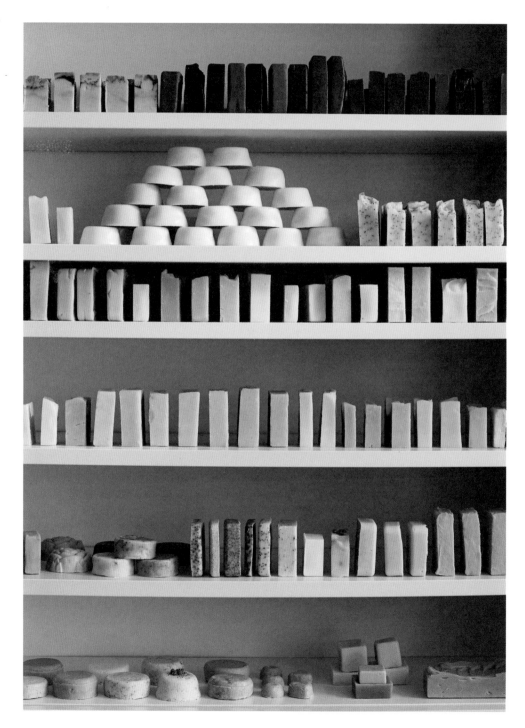

contents

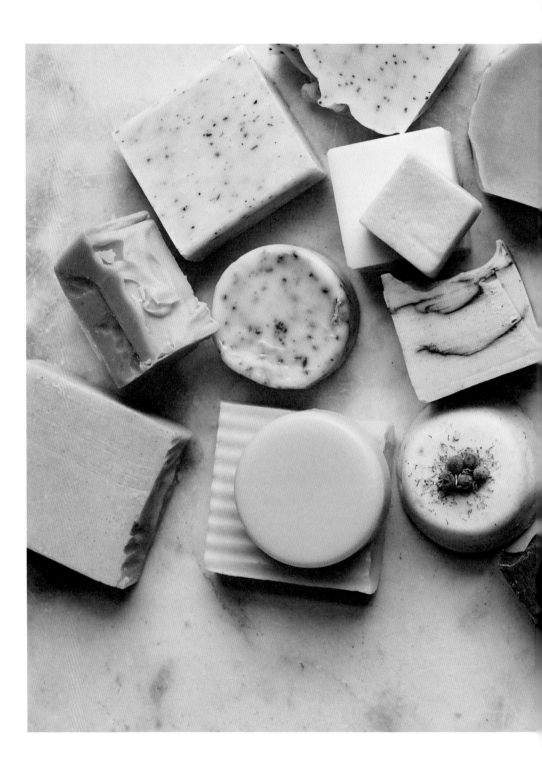

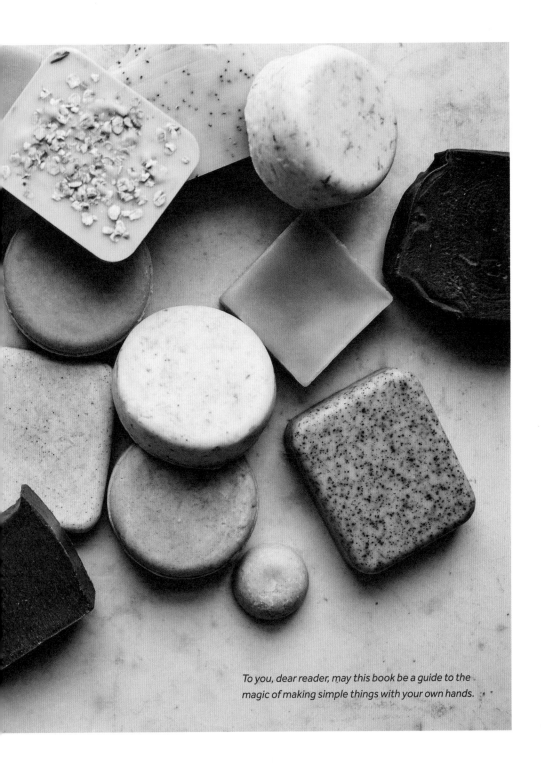

To you, dear reader, may this book be a guide to the magic of making simple things with your own hands.

introduction

It all started with soap...

Making your own personal care products at home can be one of the most empowering skills you can acquire in your life. Most people who decide to embark on a journey toward sustainable living talk about a specific moment in their life when an event, apparently very simple, struck them so much that it made them reconsider their lifestyle. My life-changing event happened to me back in 2018, when I found myself swimming in a sea of plastic bags in my kitchen. I had just moved to a new apartment in London and I was rearranging my kitchen cupboard, unpacking pasta bags to fit cuter containers. I clearly remember feeling shocked about the amount of waste plastic I had created. I then headed over to declutter the bathroom of all those plastic bath and beauty products that I had brought with me, most of which I hadn't even known I had. I clearly remember turning a bottle and reading the ingredients – I didn't even understand a single one of them. That's when it hit me: how can we live our lives without even knowing where our waste goes and without having the slightest clue of what ingredients we are putting on our skin?

My first swap was – a soap bar. At first I reused some old bars that I had lying around the house, until I realized I had no idea how a soap was made. Again, how was that possible! As a naturally curious person I had to learn. On browsing the Internet I found a few videos and, for the first time, I witnessed the soap-making reaction. It was the closest thing to magic I had ever seen. My first soap was made using just two oils: olive oil and coconut oil. I was able to create something apparently so simple yet so powerful from my kitchen, with just two oils! I remember the smell of this first soap because, after more than two years, I still have some bars left and they have retained their sweet, herbal scent, thanks to the addition of lavender essential oil to the recipe. That simplicity and minimalism has accompanied me during the formulation of all of my recipes, which I love to keep as straightforward as possible.

From there I decided to experiment with soap making using only natural ingredients. I quickly realized that there was a world of possibilities out there, but what made me happiest was to use only natural colours, botanical ingredients and essential oils – and I stood in complete awe every time the saponification reaction turned an ingredient into what was sometimes a very unexpected colour. The ingredient that shocked me the most was alkanet root, which, when infused in oil, turns it into a deep ruby red colour. When you start adding the main ingredient that turns oil into soap – sodium hydroxide – the colour of the oil morphs into a deep night blue. It holds this beautiful colour until it starts to solidify and fully become soap, at which point it turns either a fairy-like lavender-grey or a deep purple – although there are a few tricks to follow to achieve the colour you want; it is really unpredictable! That's when I realized that soap making was pretty close to wizardry.

From soap making I got more and more interested in how to use natural ingredients, and I started making most of my bath and beauty products at home and stopped buying the old single-use

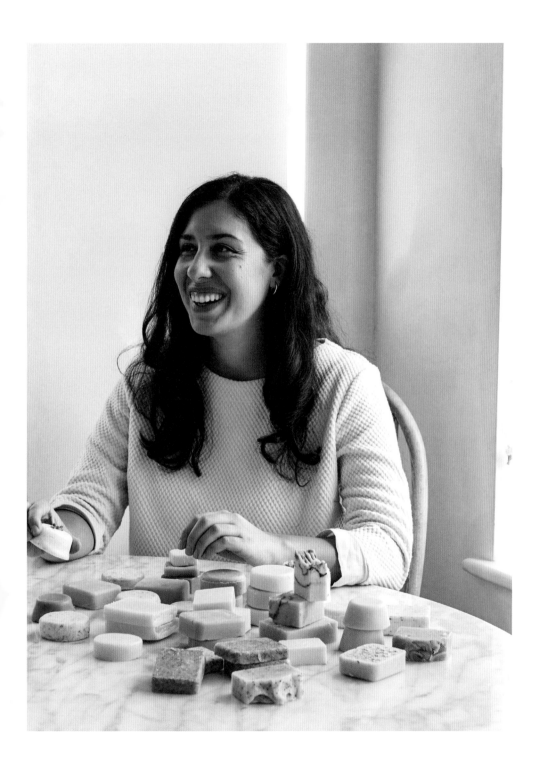

alternatives I was previously using. I also started sharing my journey and my recipes through my Instagram account, @bottegazerowaste, in an attempt to help and inspire others to live more naturally and reduce waste. I firmly believe that making your own products and starting your journey towards a more sustainable and zero-waste life should be a beautiful experience, accessible to all. However, before we start, I want you to remember a few important things:

always remember that a journey towards zero waste and natural, sustainable living is an imperfect one. Instead of striving to be perfect, respect and embrace this concept. Every single small action and effort counts more than trying to be 'perfectly zero waste' like you might see on a social media platform – this is a utopia that does not exist. What exists are small, imperfect daily steps toward a more sustainable present and future.

we all lead very different lives and have access to different resources. What works for you might not work for me or for someone else. Always build your very own zero-waste journey without comparing it to that of someone else.

don't rush, but rather enjoy the journey and its slow progress. This book has been created specifically so you have a manual to go to every time you are ready for a new adventure, or a new change. You can try out each recipe at your own pace – whether that's one every so often, or many within a short time span.

always remember that many objects have a very long lifespan. Try to reuse containers that you already have rather then buying new ones for your handmade recipes. Zero waste and natural living does not mean plastic-free; it means reusing things you already own, reducing your consumption to products you truly cherish, and refusing to buy single-use objects. One of the best containers I have is an old upcycled plastic container that once held nail polish remover pads, which I refill with my homemade salves and deodorants.

there are a few things that I don't make. I do not believe that DIYing everything is the solution because there are certain products that require specific testing in order to be safe to use. One example is sunscreen: there is no way to determine the SPF of a homemade suncream, so I recommend that you do not attempt to make your own at home – it is safer to purchase it. Another product I don't make is toothpaste. Correctly cleaning and protecting the teeth requires a lot of technical and medical knowledge, so it is safer to buy a natural, low-waste toothpaste from a reliable, tested brand.

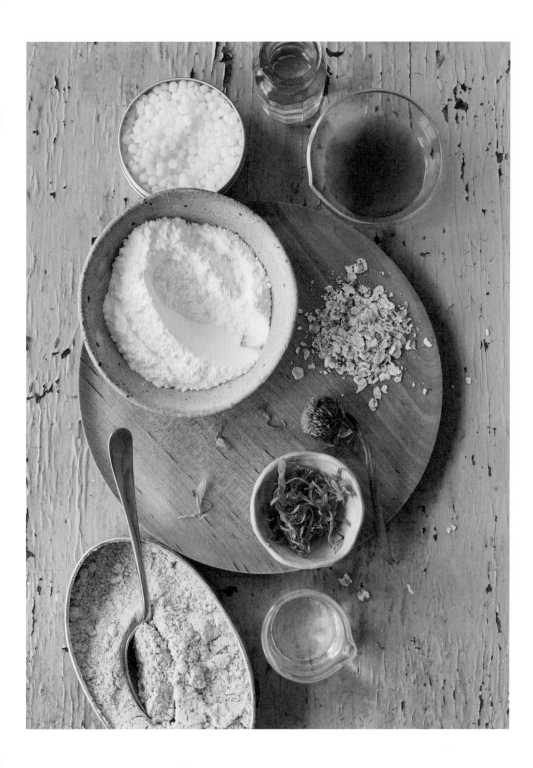

how to use this book

This book has been created to give you the simplest tools, ingredients and steps to create all the products you will need to switch to a completely natural and zero-waste routine. I have structured it in two parts: the first part explores the key ingredients and tools you will need to get started, while in the second part you will find all the recipes, further divided into four main sections: Bodycare, Skin, Soap and Haircare.

The book is illustrated throughout and each recipe has information on difficulty level, how much a recipe will make, shelf life and any safety information to be aware of.

understanding the recipes

The introduction to each recipe contains a brief description of the function of each ingredient, which also makes it easier to swap an ingredient with another one. The list of ingredients includes the weight or amount required of each ingredient and also what percentage of the recipe it equates to, which will help you when scaling up or down. Some ingredient lists are presented in the form of a chart, with the following headings:

phase: Some of the recipes have different phases – A, B, C, etc. – which you will work through in order. The ingredients that will be weighed and mixed for each phase are grouped together.

ingredient name: This column gives the common name of each ingredient.

INCI: This stands for International Nomenclature of Cosmetic Ingredients, and this column of the chart gives the universal scientific name of the ingredient, sometimes in Latin so that it is recognizable in any country no matter what language is spoken. This will help you to be sure you have the correct ingredient.

percentage: The percentage of each ingredient is given to make it easier to scale the recipe up or down, so you can make more or less of the product.

grams/ounces: These columns give you the exact amount of each ingredient needed to make the amount of product specified at the start of the recipe.

substitutions

In some recipes you may want to substitute something similar for one of the ingredients. If this is possible, the recipe will have a list of possible substitutions. Do not swap an ingredient if you are unsure – the pH of an ingredient, the function and the recommended usage rate can all vary, so swapping cosmetic ingredients is really not straightforward at all. Every time you want to make a substitution, consider the following:

- For handmade creams and haircare recipes, check that the pH of the ingredient is within the correct range of 4–6. If not, you might need to adjust the pH, which is a very advanced technique not covered in this book.

- Swapped ingredients should have the same consistency and be added in the same proportion – it's okay to swap a solid ingredient with another solid ingredient, but not replace a soft butter with a brittle butter.

- Swapping ingredients will give the product a different property, so the final effect will not be the same as before.

Are you ready? Let's get started!

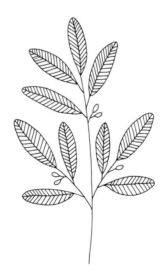

ingredients

In this book I use 10 key ingredients. Zero-waste living means simplifying your life, and finding key ingredients that can be used to make different products is one way to do that. I have selected natural ingredients that are easy to find, plastic-free and can be used to create a wide range of simple zero-waste skincare and bathroom products. The spotlight section on page 16 gives you more information on oils and butters, explaining how these two amazing categories of ingredient are normally used in a recipe and giving some examples from each category. You will soon learn how to use them to achieve nourishment, body and texture in your products – and the spotlight list will also help you to swap oils easily in a recipe, where this is possible.

Understanding the ingredients in your recipe is important, not only to know what you are putting on your skin but also to understand how these ingredients interact with each other to help create a final product. This is essential to keep recipes very simple – to avoid having too many ingredients (and more waste) – yet very effective. At the end of this section I explore how to source ingredients, using low-waste methods as much as possible.

oils

Let's start with oils. Oils are perfect to use as part of a recipe or on their own. When used alone they can replace a moisturizer and make-up remover. In fact, oil has the ability to dissolve oil, so massaging your skin with oil is a great way to get rid of any impurities, dirt and make-up. There are so many different oils that are suitable for different skin types, (see page 18).

butters

Butters are a must if you are thinking of producing your own natural and zero-waste bath and beauty products. They are packed with vitamins and fatty acids, which are great to soften dry skin, plus they make zero-waste solid products – solid! You really only need two kinds of butter: shea butter and cocoa butter. Apparently similar, they are actually very different – you can learn more about them on page 19.

waxes and emulsifying waxes

Waxes are used to give extra hardness in a solid, completely unpackaged product that you do not want to melt at high temperatures – such as a solid lip balm – or products that require a bit of stickiness, such as a body balm. Beeswax is the easiest wax to source and to work with, because it produces very stable products with excellent viscosity. My favourite plant-based wax is soy wax because it can be used to make both solid beauty products and candles, plus it's white so it's perfect if you want to play around with colours. However, it has a much lower melting point than beeswax. If you are looking for a harder vegan wax then I recommend candelilla wax.

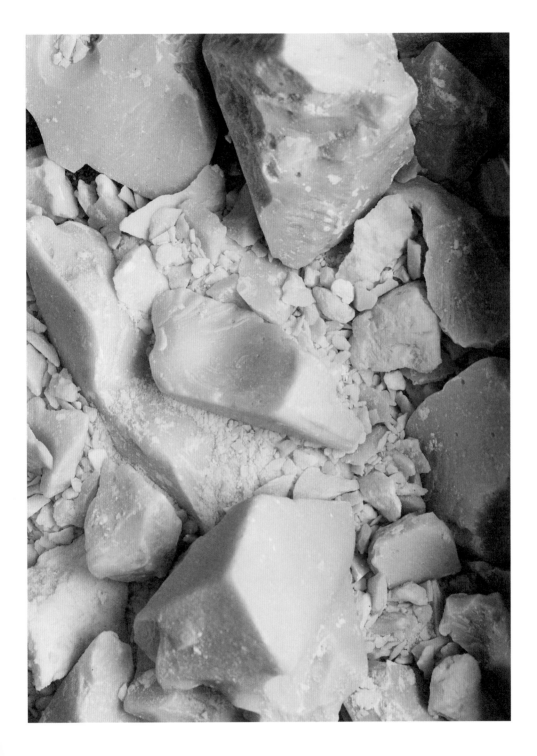

Emulsifying waxes are a somewhat different category of ingredient as they are less sticky and tacky compared to natural waxes. They are normally obtained from naturally derived ingredients such as coconut oil or rapeseed oil but they can also be derived from palm oil, which is hard to avoid in these kinds of ingredients (see page 17 for more information on palm oil). The purpose of emulsifying waxes is to allow oil and water to mix, so they are particularly useful in the creation of water-based recipes such as for handmade creams.

essential oils

Essential oils are very concentrated plant extracts that capture a plant's essence and scent. Since they are very strong compounds you should always research the maximum allowed quantities, depending on the type of essential oil and product. Please note the some essential oils might not be safe to use when pregnant and you should always check with a health provider before using. If you have a particular condition you are concerned about please check first with the supplier before using. The essential oils that I use most often in my recipes are lavender, tea tree and sweet orange.

botanical additives

Plant extracts, dried plants, roots and clays can be used to give extra purifying properties to your products or to colour and decorate products such as soaps, shampoo bars, conditioner bars or lip balms. Clays are great to use for the creation of face or hair masks; they are full of minerals and have great cleansing and detoxifying properties. They can also be used in shampoo bars to thicken the product and gently cleanse the scalp. Starches are used in recipes to help thicken products such as bath bombs, and to absorb moisture, as in deodorants. They can also be used to make a product such as a body butter less greasy. Some examples are arrowroot powder or cornflour (corn starch).

sodium hydroxide

This is a very caustic ingredient that must be handled with care; it is also sometimes called caustic soda or lye. It is an essential ingredient for making soap, and will be used in all the soap-making recipes in this book.

iron oxides

Iron oxides are naturally occurring mineral deposits, but the natural form may contain traces of heavy metals – for this reason they are heavily regulated and the form used in cosmetics is made in a laboratory and is synthetic.

surfactants

This category of ingredient is used in a wide variety of cosmetic formulations. Some surfactants pull off dirt and clean, others attract moisture and can be used to condition the hair. There are different types: some are more eco-friendly; some are milder; some are solid; some are liquid. The recipes in this book use surfactants that are eco-friendly, naturally derived and biodegradable.

deodorants

Among deodorizing ingredients we find bicarbonate of soda (baking soda) and magnesium hydroxide powder. Bicarbonate of soda is a natural deodorant and abrasive ingredient so it's perfect to use in deodorant and recipes for whitening. Due to its high pH (9) it is essential that it be used in very small quantities in order to avoid skin irritation or excessive abrasion. Some people are very sensitive to it, but it is easily replaced with magnesium hydroxide powder, which also controls sweat and odour but is more suitable for delicate skin.

preservatives and antioxidants

Preservatives are essential in products that either contain water or will come in contact with water to avoid fungi and bacteria from forming. Examples of eco-friendly preservatives are benzyl alcohol and dehydroacetic acid. Vitamin E is a powerful antioxidant that does not keep germs and bacteria away but will help to keep oils fresh.

notes:

When looking for a preservative online, make sure to use the INCI name because preservatives are often sold under different trade names which might not be included here.

I personally use preservative Geogard 221 / Cosgard for creams and shampoo bars, and Euxyl PE9010 is also an excellent broad-spectrum preservative suitable for creams, shampoo bars and conditioner bar recipes. In the US and Canada, Liquid Germall™Plus is widely available and suitable to use in creams and shampoo bars, while Optiphen™Plus would be a good option for solid conditioner bars.

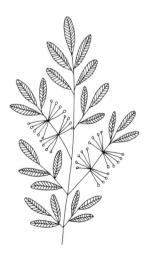

oils and butters spotlight

oils

There are so many wonderful oils available, so how do you choose? First of all, you need to consider the comedogenic scale: on a scale from 0 to 5, this is based on the absorption rate of an oil and the likelihood that it will clog your pores. You will also need to be aware of the oil's shelf life, and any contraindications (see table on page 18).

hemp seed oil

This is a very dry oil that is ideal for oily, acne prone, combination and sensitive skin. It's perfect to nourish damaged hair without weighing it down and to soothe a sensitive scalp.

grapeseed oil

A widely available and affordable oil with amazing skin softening properties, it is obtained by the seeds of grapes as a by-product of the wine industry.

jojoba

Jojoba is actually a liquid wax and not an oil. It is a temporary occlusive moisturizer, so it helps prevent moisture loss from the skin without clogging its pores, making it perfect for dry skin. In haircare recipes it's perfect for dry ends and flaky scalp – in fact, it moisturizes without clogging the scalp's pores, while keeping the oil production balanced. **Contraindications:** always store at cold temperatures because in a cold temperature/fridge it will solidify into a wax form.

sweet almond oil

This oil is very high in oleic acid, which is a monounsaturated omega-9 fatty acid known to be excellent for dry and sensitive skin. It's used in many DIY beauty recipes because it's perfect for dry and sensitive skin, but it's also lightweight and with a fairly fast absorption rate compared to, let's say, olive oil. **Contraindications:** not suitable if you suffer from a nut allergy.

castor oil

Castor oil has one of the lowest comedogenic ratings, meaning it is less likely to clog pores. It also has a very low absorption rate, making it perfect for oily/acne prone skin types. It makes an excellent base for a make-up remover or to give shine and gloss to lip balm recipes. **Contraindications:** do not use during pregnancy as it may induce contractions.

coconut oil

Coconut oil is a must-have if you want to make your own products to reduce waste. Because of its antibacterial and cleansing action it's perfect to use for deodorants or even dishwashing soap. It's one of the few oils that is solid at room temperature so it's a great candidate if you want a solid product. However, coconut oil has a high comedogenic rating, so it should not be used on the face regularly because it may clog pores. It is absorbed slower than other oils and likes to sit on the skin, so it's great if you want to add protection and moisture to your body or give a bit of shimmer and shine effect to a product like a lip balm.

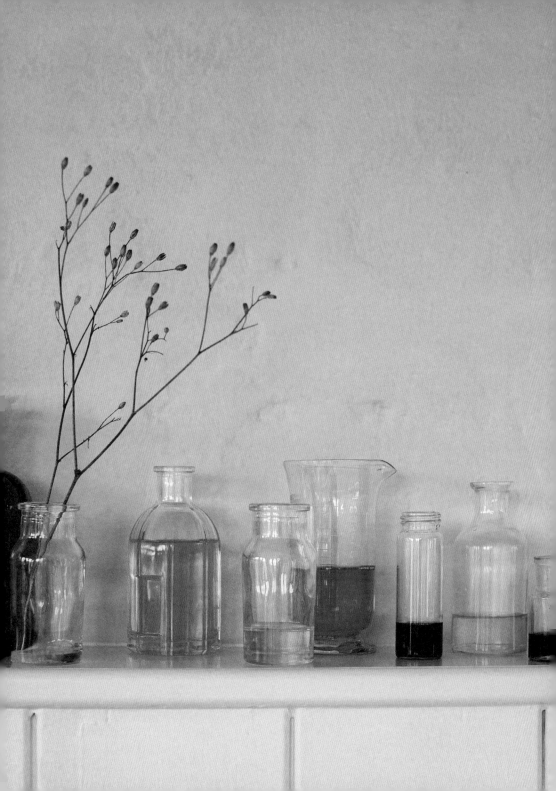

oils spotlight chart

comedogenic: 0–5 where 0 has the lowest likelihood to clog your pores and 5 the highest.
heat stable: it can be included in heated stages of formulations.

*	do not use if pregnant
**	recommended for haircare recipes
(F)	keep refrigerated
+	not suitable for nut allergies
†	also good for pets and insect repellent
‡	must be heated gently

Ingredient	Combi-nation	Oily	Acne	Dry/Sensitive	Mature	Comed-ogenic	Absorption	Heat stable	Shelf life
Apricot kernel oil	•			•		2	Fast	Yes	1 year
Argan oil**		•	•	•		0	Average	Yes	2-3 years
Avocado oil**				•	•	3	Slow	Yes	1 year
Broccoli seed oil**		•	•	•	•	1	Slow	Yes	1 year
Black seed oil*				•	•	2	Slow	Yes	1-2 years
Camellia seed**	•	•	•	•	•	1	Average	Yes	1 year
Castor oil* **		•	•			0	Slow	Yes	1 year
Cocoa butter				•		4	Average	Yes	2 years
Coconut oil				•		4	Average	Yes	2 years
Evening primrose oil				•	•	2	Fast	No	1 year
Flaxseed linseed oil**					•	4	Fast	No	6 months (F)
Grapeseed oil	•	•	•	•	•	1	Average	Yes	3-6 months (F)
Hemp seed oil**	•	•	•		•	0	Fast	No	6-12 months (F)
Jojoba (liquid wax) **	•		•	•		2	Average	Yes	2-5 years
Neem oil*†		•		•		2	Slow	Yes	1 year
Mango butter				•	•	2	Average	Yes	1 year
Olive oil				•	•	2	Slow	Yes	1–2 years
Safflower/thistle oil		•	•		•	0	Fast	Yes	1 year
Shea butter				•	•	0	Slow	Yes‡	2 years
Sunflower oil	•			•		2	Average	Yes	1 year
Sea buckthorn oil				•	•	1	Average	No	2 years
Sweet almond oil	•			•		2	Average	Yes	1 year
Tamanu oil+			•	•		2	Average	Yes	2 years
Tomato seed oil**			•	•	•	2	Average	Yes	1 year
Rice bran oil	•			•	•	2	Average	Yes	2 years
Rosehip oil	•	•	•	•	•	1	Fast	No	6-24 months

butters

There are many different types of butter, although I have found that shea butter and cocoa butter are enough to make a very wide range of products. They have very different consistencies: shea butter is softer and stickier, while coconut butter is harder and more brittle. They both have high melting points so can be combined with waxes to increase their melting point and obtain solid products that don't require packaging. When choosing a butter, always consider its scent. Shea butter has a strong rubbery scent that some people do not like; I don't mind it but often mask it a little with essential oils. Unrefined cocoa butter has a really deep chocolate smell that is delicious – but will mask the scent of any essential oils you may want to add. However, both these oils are available in a deodorized refined version that has been treated to remove the smell.

shea butter

Shea butter is packed with vitamin E and is a natural moisturizer that's perfect for dry, sensitive and eczema-prone skin. It has a very high melting point of 31° to 38°C (89° to 100°F), so it's particularly good for solid recipes where you want to keep some softness but don't want the mixture to melt, and it also adds slip, texture and stickiness. Do not use shea butter if you have a nut allergy, as it is extracted from the nut of the African shea tree. A good alternative would be mango butter, although this has a lower melting point of about 32°C (90°F).

cocoa butter

This butter is also very moisturizing, but since it's so much harder than shea butter it's excellent to use in recipes where you need the final product to be hard – like in a shampoo bar or a solid lotion. It has a melting point of 34° to 38°C (93° to 100°F).

buying ingredients

Depending on which country you live in, most supermarkets or bulk stores will carry some of the ingredients you will need – particularly those also used for cooking, such as olive oil, sunflower oil, coconut oil, avocado oil, starches and bicarbonate of soda (baking soda). Many also offer package-free ingredients used in DIY skincare, such as cocoa butter, arrowroot powder or cornflour (corn starch), extra virgin olive oil and coconut oil. Any ingredient not available locally will likely be available from an online cosmetic supplier, and I have included a list of suppliers on pages 139–140.

assessing quality

In order to assess the quality of ingredients you need to consider several different factors.

INCI (International Nomenclature of Cosmetic Ingredients)

Cosmetic ingredients should be named using their standard scientific name, which is in Latin. Sometimes ingredients are blended together to create more complex ingredients and rebranded using a different name. In that case you can check the INCI name of each ingredient to understand exactly what you are purchasing.

batch number and expiry date

These should always be clearly marked on the ingredient or product you are buying. Always check the expiry date and take this into consideration when formulating a product.

manufacturing methods

An organically-farmed ingredient will be higher quality but will also be way more expensive. It is up to you to decide whether you want to invest in organic ingredients; it will also depend a lot on the kind of product you want to make. Certifications are one way to assess the quality and control of the supply chain of an ingredient, but might vary by country. Every certification has standards that the manufacturer must adhere to in order to achieve certification. However, an ingredient without an organic certificate is not necessarily a fake – it may not have formal certification but could still be organic or Fair Trade. Not all ingredients can be organic – for example, you will not find an organic bicarbonate of soda (baking soda)!

Another way to determine the quality of an ingredient is by its method of extraction, and this is particularly useful for oils and butters. The highest quality oils are normally CO_2 extracted, followed by cold pressed, because these methods do not use high heat or chemical solvents and therefore preserve the oil's qualities. You can also check if an oil has been left unrefined or has been deodorized and/or bleached. Some oils are refined to remove their impurities and improve their shelf life, while deodorizing and bleaching is applied to remove scent or strong colour. The choice is yours, depending on which product you want to make; however, generally speaking, an oil left raw and unrefined is more expensive and contains more of those nutrients that might have got lost in oils that have gone through a refinement process.

data sheets

If you want to learn more about an ingredient, your supplier should be able to provide a Certificate of Analysis (COA) and Material Safety Data Sheet (MSDS), or an International Fragrance Association (IFRA) Certificate for essential oils and fragrances. Additionally, many cosmetic supplier websites contain usage guidance on the maximum quantities recommended for the ingredient they are selling.

supply chain

This information will be useful to assess if an ingredient has been manufactured using specific ethical standards. For example, Fair Trade means that an ingredient has been manufactured by workers who are paid fairly. Vegan means that the ingredient does not include animal products, but does not necessarily mean that it has not been tested on animals. Certifications will help you to check these points, but where there is no certification I recommend checking with the suppliers. They should be able to clarify your doubts to a certain extent, depending on how direct their control on the supply chain is.

about palm oil

Palm oil comes from the fruit of palm trees and is used to make many food as well as cosmetic ingredients because it contains a mix of fatty acids with unique properties that impart incredible creaminess and viscosity to products. It is a very efficient crop – it requires less land and water compared to other crops such as soy or coconut. As a result it has been over-harvested, driving its price down and increasing demand, which raised the need for more palm oil crops. This in turn led to deforestation in exploited areas, also endangering animal species such as the orangutan, pygmy elephant and Sumatran rhino.

This is a controversial topic, but something that is essential to consider because eventually you will encounter recipes where it will be difficult or impossible to source palm oil-free alternatives to certain ingredients. This is partly because such ingredients simply might not be available or easy to source where you live, or because palm oil exists within a compound but is labelled as vegetable oil – suppliers often do not disclose exactly which vegetable oils have been used in the manufacturing of a specific ingredient. Organizations such as the Roundtable on Sustainable Palm Oil (RSPO) strive to provide a global standard for sustainably sourced palm oil, but many ingredients do not carry this certification so it is difficult to know if the palm oil has been sourced sustainably or not. Another thing to consider is that some palm-free alternatives are not necessarily more sustainable than palm-derived ingredients – they may come from a crop that requires way more water or more land. The issue of palm oil is very complex and the cosmetic industry has a lot of work to do to create palm oil-free alternatives. So if you are unable to source a palm oil-free ingredient, don't feel ashamed or let this put you off; it really is all about finding a balance and, most importantly, buying from reputable suppliers.

packaging and ingredient storage

While sadly the most common packaging method is still plastic, certain suppliers do carry smaller quantities of ingredients – such as oils or essential oils – packaged in glass or aluminium. Some suppliers will be more flexible than others and will agree to send ingredients like solid butters in paper. For security reasons this will not always be possible, but if you think this might be an option for a certain ingredient it is always worth asking.

If you are unable to find an ingredient plastic-free, my recommendation is to purchase it in a larger quantity; this is exactly the concept behind bulk stores – they are able to lower their environmental impact by purchasing large amounts of produce in big plastic containers, to then resell smaller quantities to consumers in reusable or compostable packaging. Now, this does not necessarily mean you need to go out and buy 5 litres (9 pints) of sweet almond oil, but if you know you will use this oil in many different recipes it is worth purchasing a 1 litre (2 pint) plastic bottle as opposed to a small 100 millilitre (¼ pint) plastic bottle. However, when you purchase an ingredient in bulk make sure you check the ingredient's shelf life, expiry date and storage recommendations. Some ingredients have a very long shelf life of one to two years, while others will have a shelf life of only a few months and might need to be kept in the fridge.

storage of ingredients

Always store cosmetic ingredients in a clean and dry environment, keeping them in their original containers if possible to avoid contamination. Shelf life really depends on the specific ingredient, but is normally between six months and one to two years. In general, ingredients with a shelf life of six months should be stored in the fridge once opened.

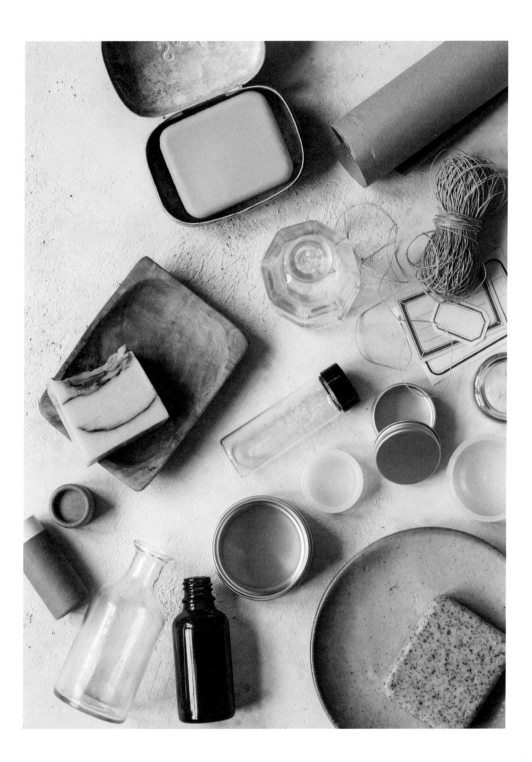

tools and equipment

In this section I explain what tools you will need to get started; don't worry, you will not require much specialized equipment and you can probably buy most things second-hand. You may even have many of the items already in your kitchen – although it's important to have a set of dedicated items for making your cosmetics and never use them for food purposes afterwards. Focus on tools that are durable and reusable; most of this equipment is available in your local supermarket, from online stores or through online cosmetic stores (see pages 139–140).

I like to categorize tools by their main function; this way, you will notice that you can use the same tools across similar projects.

HYGIENE AND SAFETY: reusable rubber gloves, mask/respirator, reusable goggles

Although this varies depending on which recipe you are working on, it is good manufacturing practice to wear a pair of rubber gloves when handling cosmetic ingredients. This not only protects your hands but also prevents you from contaminating the finished result. Tight-fitting reusable rubber gloves are best and can be cleaned – disposable ones break easily. For making soap or shampoo bars a mask or respirator will also be required to protect you from the fumes when preparing the lye solution and from the sodium cocoyl isethionate powder, which is very fine and unpleasant to breathe in. For soap making you will also need a pair of reusable goggles to protect your eyes when handling lye and raw soap; it is important that they also cover your eyes from the side.

WEIGHING AND MEASURING: bowls, weighing scale, pipettes

You will need several bowls for weighing and mixing your ingredients. Very simple small ceramic or glass bowls – you can even reuse dessert ramekins – are useful to weigh small amounts of ingredients. If you are just using the bowls to weigh the ingredients they can be of any material, but for soap making you will need heat-safe glass, stainless steel or very heavy-duty plastic bowls that can withstand temperatures up to 93°C (200°F). Never use aluminium bowls for soap making, as this metal can react with the sodium hydroxide.

Precision is an important component to consider when formulating a product – although some recipes may call for tablespoons/teaspoons, you will often need to be more precise by weighing using a scale. You can use any scale, but for more specialized projects like soap making it's best to use a high precision digital scale that does not round up the numbers. If you need to precisely measure small amounts of liquid, pipettes can be of great help. I suggest investing in a set of reusable glass pipettes with a silicone top.

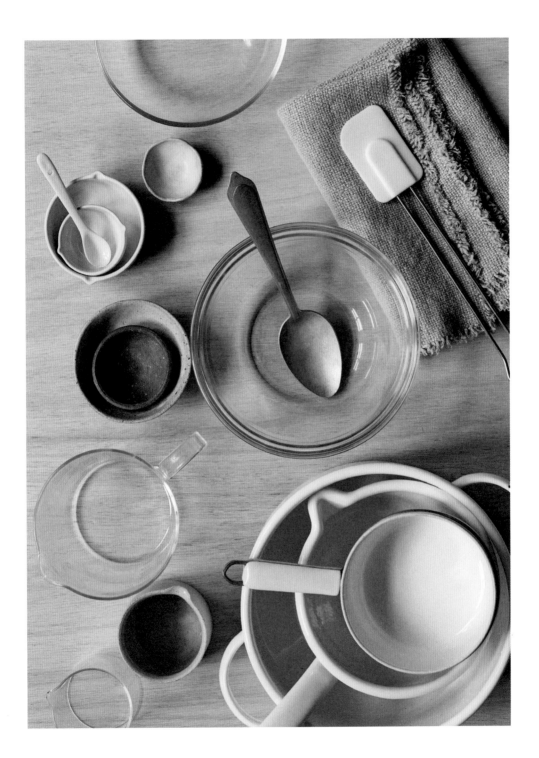

HEATING AND MELTING: thermometer, stainless steel saucepan, heat-safe jugs and bowls

The thermometer is used to measure the temperature of your ingredients when making soap or cream. The best option is a digital laser thermometer that keeps you distanced from the ingredients, or you can opt for a cheaper candy thermometer alternative (but make sure that the stick is not in aluminium).

A large stainless steel saucepan about 15cm (6in) in diameter, and heat-safe ceramic stainless steel or glass jugs and bowls or beakers are also perfect to melt the ingredients for many projects, weigh lye solution and mix your soap batter. You can also use the saucepan to make a bain-marie to melt ingredients gently (see page 29).

MIXING: spoons and spatulas, stick blender, electric whisk

You will need a very simple and common mixing tool: a spoon! A tablespoon and a teaspoon would work just fine – just make sure they are stainless steel, because this is a requirement for the soap-making projects. A silicone spatula is optional but is also incredibly useful: it will help you scrape out any precious ingredient residue still stuck inside your bowl so nothing goes to waste! Do not use wooden utensils because these can be damaged by the sodium hydroxide. For more specialized projects like soap making, creams and body butter you will need a stick blender and an electric whisk or milk frother. Making soap stirring with a spoon or spatula will take you hours, compared to a few seconds using a stick blender. Any low-priced, one to two-speed setting stick blender will be fine.

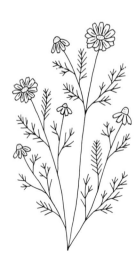

SHAPING AND STORING: jars and/or tins, moulds, non-serrated kitchen knife

For most projects you will be able to reuse old jars or tins, into which you can pour your deodorants or creams to set. However, as you will also be making lots of solid products, I suggest investing in a set of moulds in different sizes and shapes. Silicone moulds are really affordable and can be reused for a very long time, if kept with care. A muffin silicone mould with six holes, and a couple of moulds with a smaller cavity, would be perfect. You can really just unleash your creative soul and get the shape you love the most.

For soap making avoid rigid metal or plastic moulds, as you will never get the soap out after it has hardened. To start off, you could upcycle a milk carton by cutting it in half and using the base as your mould.

When you are more experienced you may want to make larger batches of soap in a wooden mould lined with greaseproof (parchment) paper, in which case you will also need a non-serrated knife to cut it into bars once it is unmoulded. Later on your soap-making journey you could also invest in a soap cutter.

tips

Although most recipes call for completely natural ingredients, many of which are also edible, I advise you to dedicate a set of equipment just for your cosmetic-making experiments.

Glass pipettes can be cleaned in the dishwasher by popping them upright on the spikes that support the plates.

Technically you could weigh all the oils in the same heat-safe container you will use to make the rest of the recipe later, but if you add a wrong amount of an oil you cannot reverse the action and you could end up with wrong quantities.

Each soap-making ingredient, whether it is liquid or solid, is always measured in weight and not by volume. This is because different oils might have very different weights even if they are of the same volume. For example, castor oil is a very heavy and thick liquid that will weigh much more than the same volume of sweet almond oil. Soap making is truly a precision game!

before you begin

These simple tips will help you achieve a successful result with your cosmetics making, and will keep you safe while you are making your products.

general safety and hygiene

A clean and tidy working environment can prevent any accidents and spills from happening, ensuring that the products you are making do not become contaminated, and that you are not injured.

- Wash your hands well with soap before manufacturing a product.

- Use clean equipment and don't mix equipment you use for food with your equipment for cosmetics.

- If possible, sterilize your equipment with 90% – or even better 99.9% – surgical spirit (rubbing alcohol).

- Work in a tidy, clean environment and keep long hair tied back.

- Cover any surfaces with towels or protective papers to protect your work area from any possible spills.

- Certain projects call for mandatory gloves, goggles and/or masks to be worn. If this is the case, it will be noted at the start of the recipe in the Safety Notes box.

- Do not use essential oils if you are pregnant – some of them can induce early contractions – and avoid them if you have sensitive skin. I also recommend that you do not use essential oils in products that will be used on children.

how to prepare a bain-marie

A bain-marie is a heated container of water in which you place heat-safe containers to gently heat and melt their contents.

1. Add 3cm (1in) of tap water into a large stainless steel saucepan and place on the stove at a very low heat.
2. In the meantime, weigh the ingredients to be melted into separate heat-safe jugs or other tall-sided containers.
3. When the water in the saucepan has started simmering, place the containers into the saucepan. Leave until the contents melt, making sure that the water in the saucepan does not boil over and contaminate the ingredients.

how to make an oil infusion

Infusing oils is a great way to add amazing properties, colours and textures to your creations – in particular lotions, balms or cold-process soap. Each oil and each spice or herb has unique properties, so you can customize the benefits added to your product depending on skin type and the scent and colour you want to achieve. You can infuse spices, such as turmeric or paprika, herbs and powders like green tea, spirulina and sandalwood, or even roots like alkanet root or madder root. They will all give beautiful, bright natural colours to your product and, depending on what herb or spice you are using, the scent will carry through the infusion leaving a very mild smell. You can also infuse an ingredient only for its properties even though it will not leave much of a colour or scent. My favourite infusions are chamomile for its calming properties or calendula for its anti-inflammatory properties. You can infuse

any type of oil that does not become solid at colder temperatures, such as coconut oil, rice bran oil, sunflower oil, rapeseed oil or sweet almond oil. One of my favourite oils to infuse is olive oil because it is a flexible oil that is gentle on the skin. I use it in large percentages in my cold-process soaps. There are different infusion methods you can follow; here are three of the most popular ones.

natural infusion method

This first method involves letting the chosen ingredient sit in the oil for around two to four weeks, so that the oil absorbs all the beneficial properties of the herb. The quantity of ingredient to use will depend on what ingredient you are infusing and how much oil you want to infuse. For spices a good starting ratio is two teaspoons of your chosen spice, powder or root into 100g (3.5oz) of oil. For herbs like rosemary, four to five twigs would be sufficient, while for flowers like calendula and chamomile, fill the jar halfway and then fill up with oil.

sun infusion method

The sun infusion method involves using the sun as a source of heat for two to four weeks. The benefit from using a sun infusion is that the heat from the sun can speed up the infusion process while preserving the beneficial plant properties, which might otherwise be weakened in the heat-induced method.

heat induced method

This method is perfect if you are in a rush because it is fast and easy, but the infusion might lose some of the characteristics of the oils and herbs. Put the same proportions of herb and oil in a mason jar, and then place the jar in a saucepan filled with water. Place on the stove and leave to simmer for 40 minutes over very low heat. I recommend doing several infusions at the same time to offset the energy usage of this method.

filtering out the infusion

Once your infusion is ready, you can either filter the deposit out to benefit just from the infused oil properties and colour, or keep the deposit in for extra exfoliating properties. Spices will normally sink to the bottom of the jar, so to keep some in the infusion you can gently pour the oil leaving the residue on the bottom. However, remember that keeping a lot of deposit in an infusion might make your final product more prone to spoilage. If you want to filter out the deposit, fix a piece of cheesecloth or an old stocking onto the mouth of the jar and pour the oil into a separate bowl or container, using a funnel if the opening is not very wide.

precision and labelling

When working with cosmetic ingredients it is important to be as precise as possible. Many recipes found online call for teaspoons or tablespoons, but it is good practice to start measuring quantities in grams or ounces or, even better, by a percentage of the ingredients required. If you use percentages you will be able to understand how a product is formulated, and you will also be able to resize the recipe very easily!

Taking lots of notes during the formulation process is also very important. How did that texture turn out? Did the scent you chose come through in the final product or not? Recording everything will help you learn from any mistakes and become a better formulator.

Finally, make sure to label your products with the name, batch and the manufacturing date (for example, 'Lavender soap bar, 12 March 2024'). This way you will not confuse the product with another one, and you can keep track of the product's shelf life.

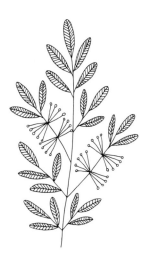

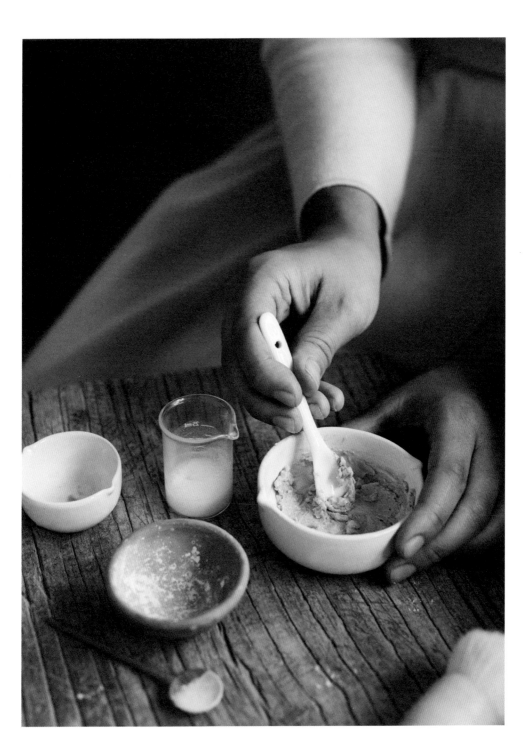

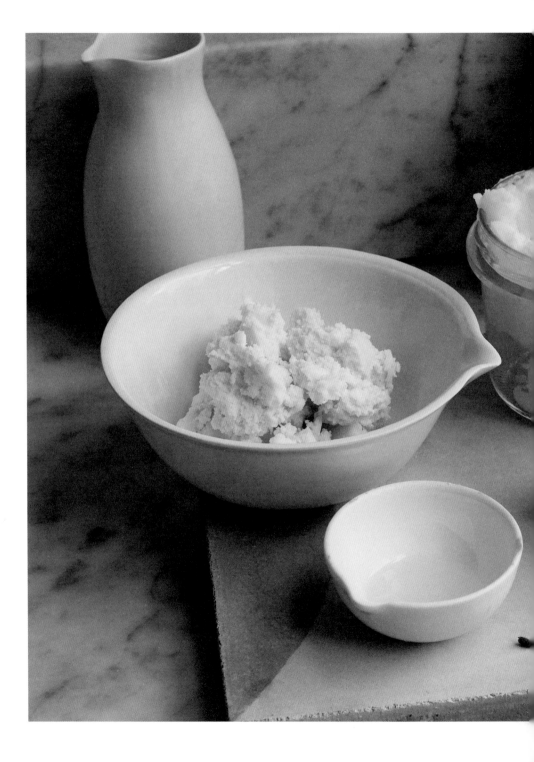

bodycare

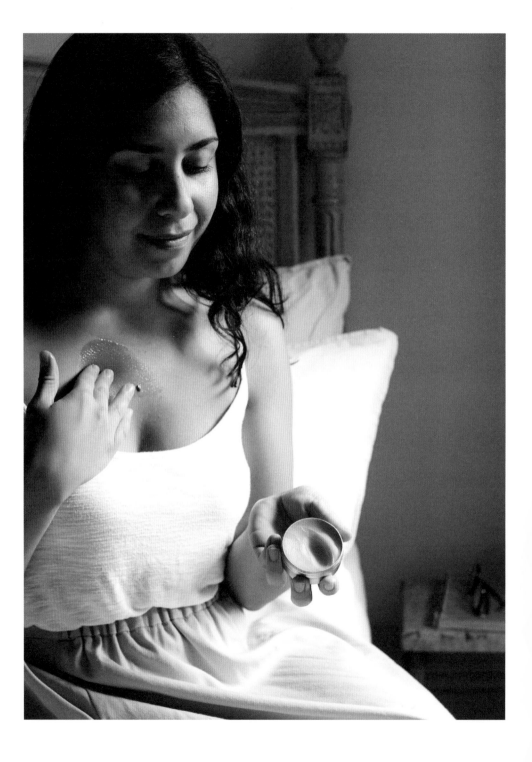

bodycare

The recipes included in this section contain very few ingredients – but you will soon notice that they are incredibly effective. Adopting a zero-waste bodycare routine will also open the doors to more natural remedies that rely mostly on the power of very few plant-based ingredients.

One of my favourite recipes is for my handmade deodorant, which contains only five ingredients. Since making this recipe for the first time many years ago, I have never looked back. I normally apply deodorant first thing in the morning right after I take a shower, but it can be applied a second time later in the day if needed. Thanks to the use of shea butter this deodorant does not melt very easily, even at high temperatures. I like to carry a tin of it with me when I am on the go, so I can re-apply it in the middle of the day in the office on a very hot day, or after a gym workout.

Something I like to use during both winter and summer months is a fluffy whipped body butter, so this section also includes a recipe for a really rich, deeply nourishing body butter that is perfect for very dry winter hands or feet.

Before going to bed I like to immerse myself in the relaxing scent of lavender; I use it in the form of a herbal body salve. A body salve is a soothing concoction formulated with a butter, an oil and a wax, which results in a rich and deeply nourishing treatment. The addition of essential oils makes it a truly therapeutic natural remedy to release tension, ease you towards sleep before going to bed, or even provide relief from muscle pain. The basic body salve recipe in this section can be used to create all kinds of interesting salves, such as a super-relaxing sleep-tight lavender-infused salve, a cooling eucalyptus salve to find relief if you have a cold, or a mosquito-repellent citronella salve.

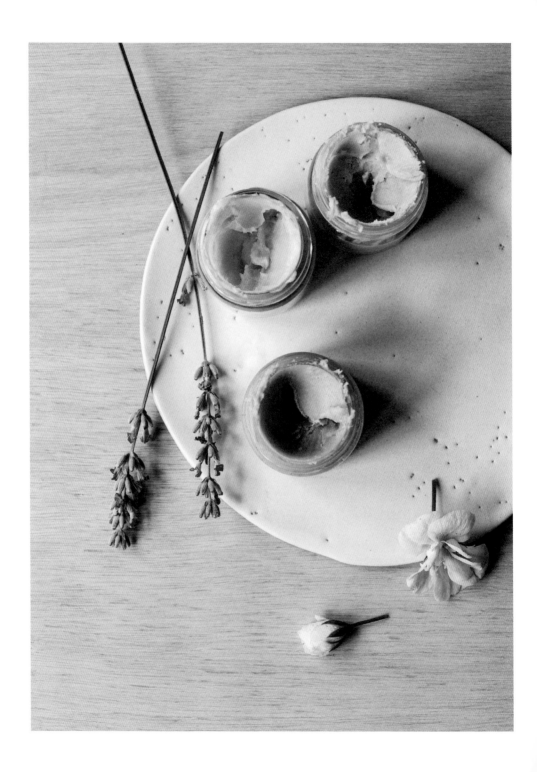

body butter

Difficulty level: Beginner
Recipe makes: 30g (1oz)
Shelf life: 6 months

You can whip butter and oils just like whipped cream to obtain an incredibly fluffy body butter. What's best is that you really can do it with just two ingredients: a butter and an oil. The texture of this body butter is really decadent and quite oily, so it is perfect for very dry winter hands, dry feet or to use as a post-shaving or post-shower body lotion. If you want to make this lotion a little less greasy, you can add a little bit of arrowroot powder or cornflour (corn starch), or alternatively a lightweight clay such as pink clay or kaolin clay.

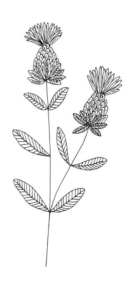

ingredients

- 50% soft butter, such as raw, unrefined shea butter: 15g (0.53oz)
- 50% oil, such as hemp seed oil: 15g (0.53oz)
- Optional additives: ½ teaspoon arrowroot powder or cornflour (corn starch), 1 drop vitamin E and 2–3 drops of essential oil(s) – I used lavender and geranium essential oils

equipment

- High precision scales
- Heat-safe bowl
- Stainless steel saucepan
- Tablespoon
- Whisk (if possible electric but a hand whisk or a fork is fine)
- 30g (1oz) wide-mouthed aluminium or glass jar with lid, or upcycled plastic jar

safety notes

Because this lotion does not contain water, it does not need a preservative and has a shelf life of about six months. A little goes a very long way! If you are using an oil with a short shelf life, for example hemp seed or grapeseed oil, I recommend adding a drop of vitamin E to help slow down the oxidation process (this is when the oil goes rancid).

substitutions

For the oil part you can choose any oil you want, depending on the intended usage – for instance, if you want to use it on your face, coconut oil may not be the best choice as it has a comedogenic score of 4. But it is perfectly fine if you plan to use this lotion only on the hands or body.

If you are also planning to use this lotion on the face, I would recommend using a lightweight oil with a low comedogenic rating of 0 –2 – for instance, grapeseed, safflower or sweet almond oil, or even a high quality sunflower oil. You could also combine different oils together or infuse the oil with a botanical element, such as calendula petals or chamomile flowers, to give it very soothing properties. I like to use a mix of grapeseed oil and hemp seed oil for use on the face/body, or sweet almond oil. Instructions on how to prepare your own oil infusions are on page 29.

Shea butter is a great choice because it has a very low comedogenic rating of 0, which means that it will not clog your pores. Don't be tricked by its sticky and oily consistency – shea butter is great to use, especially in a lotion for the face. I use this butter whenever I feel my skin is dry, particularly after taking a shower. Shea butter is also quite easy to find plastic-free and can often be sold in paper. You can replace it with mango butter, or if you use cocoa butter the texture will be much firmer.

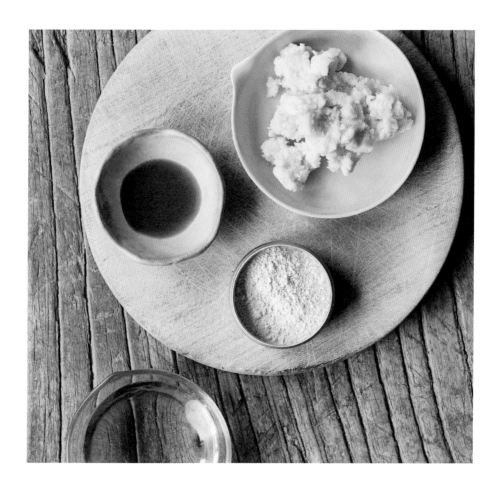

tip

For a soothing after-sun butter, use coconut oil or a lightweight oil such as safflower or sunflower, which you could infuse with calendula petals. Peppermint, rosemary or eucalyptus are all great cooling essential oils that would be perfect in an aftershave or after-sun butter.

instructions

1. Weigh out the shea butter into a bowl.

2. Add the oil to the shea butter; if you have chosen a heat-sensitive oil, such as hemp seed oil, then it is best to add the oil only after the shea butter has been melted in step 3.

3. Melt the shea butter slowly in a bain-marie (see page 29) or in the microwave, whichever option you have – although using a bain-marie is much better as sudden heat can disrupt some of the shea butter's precious nutrients.

4. Once melted, remove the bowl from the bain-marie and allow the mixture to cool down and harden in the freezer or fridge – this will make the whipping part a bit easier. It usually takes around 30 minutes in the fridge or 15 minutes in the freezer – the mixture should not be rock solid; it needs to be in a 'gel' stage between liquid and solid.

5. Remove the semi-solid mixture from the freezer or fridge. At this point you can add the optional ingredients to make the lotion better suited to your needs. Half a teaspoon of arrowroot powder or cornflour (corn starch) will make the lotion less greasy. If you have used an oil with a short shelf life – such as hemp seed oil – then you can add vitamin E, which can extend its life. Finally you could add a maximum of 2–3 drops of essential oils – I used lavender and geranium, which smell really relaxing and soothing together.

6. Once all of the ingredients are added, whip everything together to a soft and fluffy consistency. If you are making a small batch, I suggest using a small beaker and just one whisk. It should take you about 5–10 minutes to obtain a light, fluffy and soft cream-like consistency.

7. When you have your desired consistency, transfer this divine goodness into a small clean jar and enjoy! Over a few days the mixture will lose a little of the air and will become less fluffy and more buttery, but it will still be an incredible zero-waste treat for your body. If you find the butter becomes too firm, you can increase the amount of oil in the recipe to fit your needs.

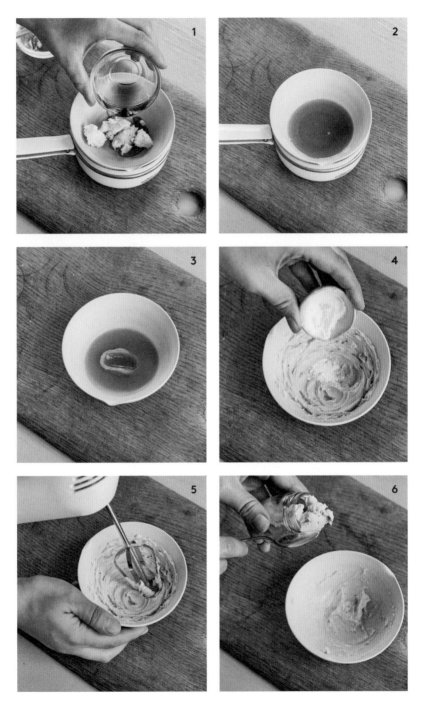

shea butter deodorant and antiperspirant

Difficulty level: Beginner
Recipe makes: 50g (1.76oz)
Shelf life: 6 months

Natural deodorant was one of the first products I made after going zero waste. This recipe is very quick and satisfying and you will only need five ingredients: shea butter, coconut oil, arrowroot powder, essential oils and bicarbonate of soda (baking soda). A great thing about this deodorant is that it does not require any wax – shea butter gives the right stickiness you want in a deodorant, but without the tackiness of a wax. This also means it will still remain hard even during the summer at fairly high temperatures, because it calls for only a little coconut oil while the shea butter has a high melting point of 31° to 38°C (89° to 100°F). The starch component will help absorb moisture so this deodorant will easily be effective for up to eight hours.

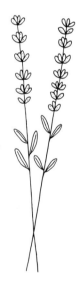

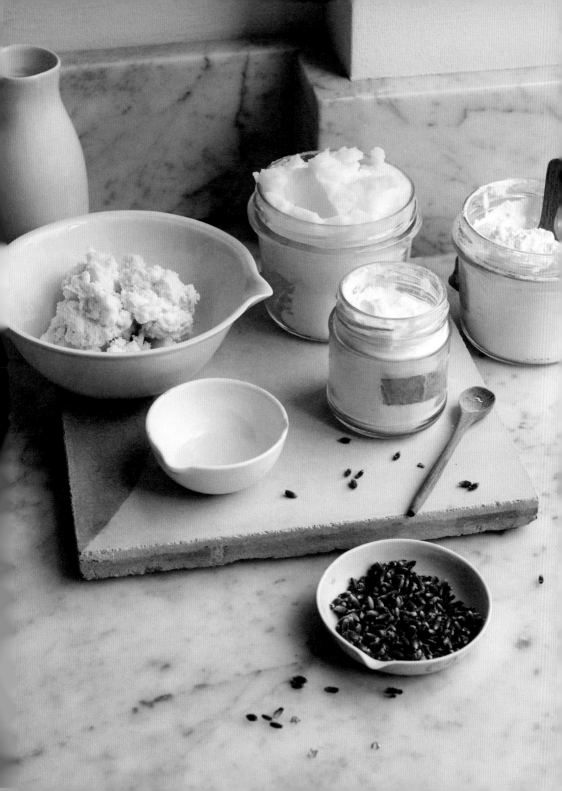

ingredients

- 63% shea butter: 31.50g (1.11oz) or 2 tablespoons
- 8% coconut oil: 4g (0.14oz) or 1 teaspoon
- 30% arrowroot powder or cornflour (corn starch): 15g (0.53oz) or 2 tablespoons
- 1% bicarbonate of soda (baking soda) or food-grade magnesium hydroxide powder: 0.5g (0.02oz)
- 1% essential oil or essential oil blend of your choice – I chose lavender: 0.5g (0.02oz) or 15 drops

equipment

- High precision scales
- Heat-safe bowl
- Stainless steel saucepan
- Tablespoon and teaspoon
- Silicone spatula (optional)
- 50g (1.76oz) wide-mouthed aluminium, glass jar with lid or upcycled plastic jar

safety notes

A little note on bicarbonate of soda (baking soda): although you will use a very small amount, this has a very alkaline pH of 9, so it may be irritating for some people's skin (I am in this category). You can substitute magnesium hydroxide instead, which will also give your deodorant a more antiperspirant effect. You can source magnesium hydroxide from food supplements websites.

I recommend lavender, tea tree, grapefruit or peppermint essential oil for this recipe. If you are using a citrus essential oil (such as lemon or grapefruit) avoid direct sun exposure as they are photosensitizing and so can burn your skin.

tip

Please note that the consistency of the deodorant will vary depending on the room temperature. If it is very hot and you feel that the deodorant is too liquid, you can add an extra tablespoon of arrowroot powder/corn flour and 1 extra tablespoon of shea butter.

If you are making this recipe when it's cold and you find it's too hard, loosen it up with your finger after having washed your hands before applying it. You can, if you want to make it softer, add more coconut oil or remove some arrowroot powder/corn flour.

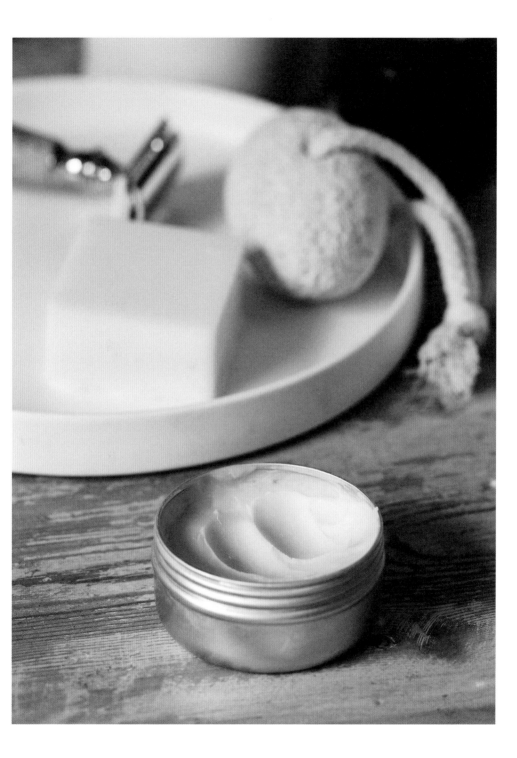

instructions

1. Weigh the shea butter and the coconut oil in a ceramic or glass heat-safe bowl.

2. Melt the shea butter along with the coconut oil in a bain-marie (see page 29) until fully melted. For this quantity, it should take you about 4–5 minutes on the stove at a low heat, or two minutes in the microwave at a medium heat. I recommend melting it in bain-marie so as not to disrupt the nutrients of the shea butter.

3. Once melted, remove the shea butter and coconut oil from the microwave or keep on the stove but turn the heat off.

4. Add the arrowroot powder or cornflour (corn starch) and bicarbonate of soda or magnesium hydroxide powder to the melted shea butter and coconut oil, and mix until everything is well incorporated and there are no clumps left.

5. Remove the bowl from the saucepan, add the essential oil and mix well.

6. Pour into a tin or a 50g (1.76oz) glass jar with a wide mouth.

7. Place in the freezer for about one hour, then take it out and let it soften down and warm up to room temperature before using it.

8. To apply, scoop up a pea-size amount with a clean finger and gently rub into your armpit until completely melted onto your skin.

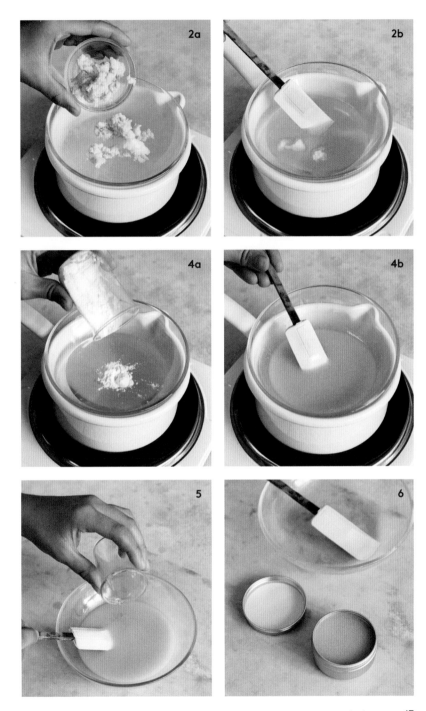

body salves

Difficulty level: Beginner
Recipe makes: 50g (1.76oz)
Shelf life: 6 months

Body salves are great to soothe your skin, and you can add the essential oil of your choice for different therapeutic effects – see the information on different essential oils overleaf.

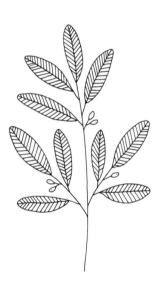

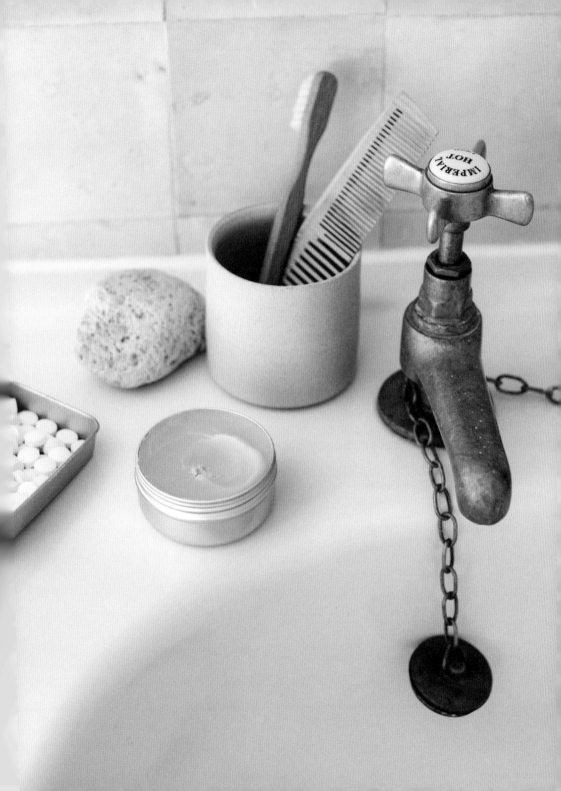

ingredients

nourishing body salve

- 40% extra virgin olive oil: 20g (0.71oz)
- 30% cocoa butter: 15g (0.53oz)
- 21% sweet almond oil: 10.50g (0.37oz)
- 8% beeswax: 4g (0.14oz)
- 1% essential oil: 0.50g (0.02oz) (optional – pick the essential oil of your choice from the Suggested essential oils list, below)

vegan soy wax body salve

- 55% sweet almond oil: 27.50g (0.97oz)
- 25% cocoa butter: 12.50g (0.44oz)
- 19% soy wax: 9.50g (0.34oz)
- 1% essential oil: 0.50g (0.02oz) (optional)

suggested essential oils

- Lavender: soothing, perfect to apply on the chest or behind the ears before a good night's sleep.
- Eucalyptus and peppermint: cooling and refreshing, ideal to apply on the chest or near the nostrils or chest if you have a cold, or on sore muscles after a workout.
- Tea tree: perfect as an anti-mosquito bite salve, apply it on the arms, legs and feet.

equipment

- High precision scales
- Heat-safe jug or bowl
- Stainless steel saucepan
- Tablespoon
- 50g (1.76oz) wide-mouthed aluminium or glass jar with lid, or upcycled plastic jar
- Silicone spatula (optional)

safety notes

This recipe uses essential oils, which are plant extracts that come with some contraindications. If you are adding them, please do not exceed 1% of the total quantity of ingredients in the recipe.

If you have sensitive skin I suggest omitting the essential oils – the products will still be deeply nourishing and effective. If you are pregnant or plan to use the salves for your children, please do not use any essential oils.

tip

If you use a low shelf-life oil such as hemp seed oil, which normally expires after about six months, I recommend including vitamin E for up to 0.5% of your recipe – for the amounts given in this recipe use 0.25g (0.01oz).

For the vegan soy wax variation, do not freeze the ingredients for more than 20 minutes because the soy wax will crack when exposed to a cold temperature for an extended period. If possible, allow to solidify at room temperature.

If you find your product turns out a bit grainy, this could be either because you did not melt the ingredients fully, or because you melted them too fast, you did not transfer them straight into the freezer. If this is the case, try to re-melt them very gently, and place the tin with the melted ingredients straight into the freezer.

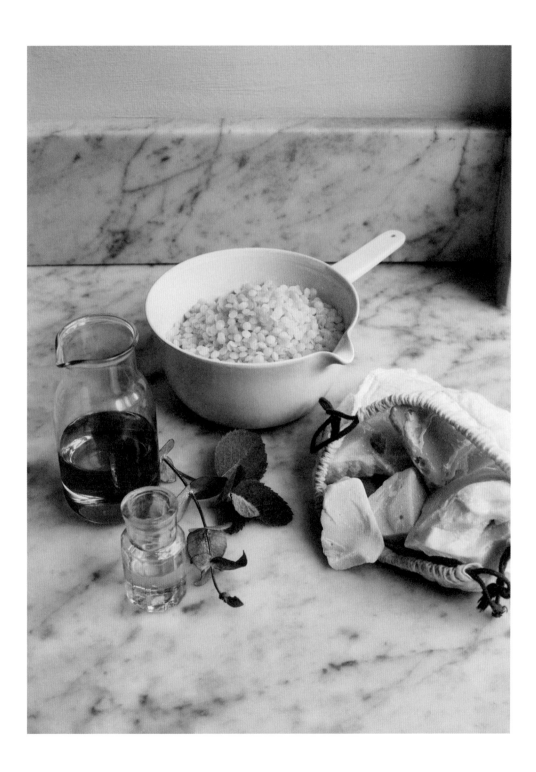

instructions

1. Weigh the oil, butter and wax into the heat-safe jug or bowl.

2. Melt these ingredients at low heat in a bain-marie (see page 29) for at least 15 minutes, mixing now and then.

3. Remove from the heat and add any essential oils and optional vitamin E.

4. Pour into your chosen container and place in the freezer for about 30 minutes to solidify.

subsitutions

You can use any other oil – avocado oil, sunflower oil, grapeseed oil, coconut oil or tomato seed oil all make great options. Check the oils spotlight chart on page 18.

If you want to give your body salve a chocolate smell, use unrefined cocoa butter. However, this will cover the smell of any essential oils.

You can use shea butter or mango butter instead of the cocoa butter, but the result will be much softer.

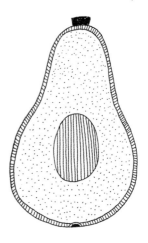

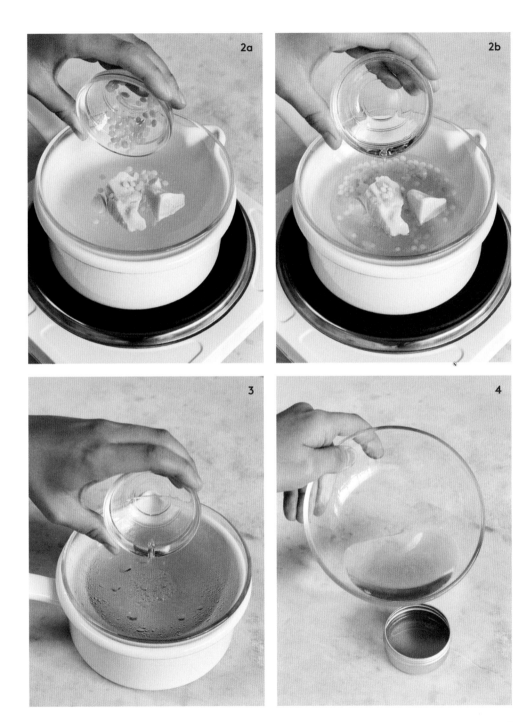

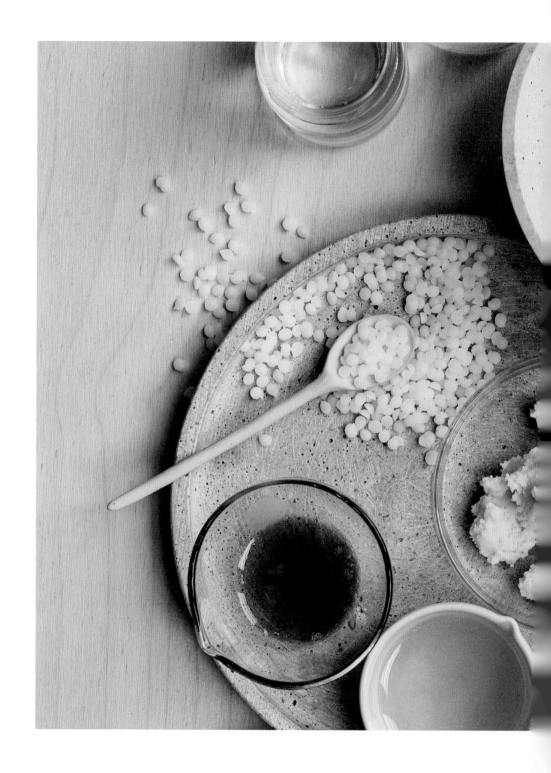

skincare

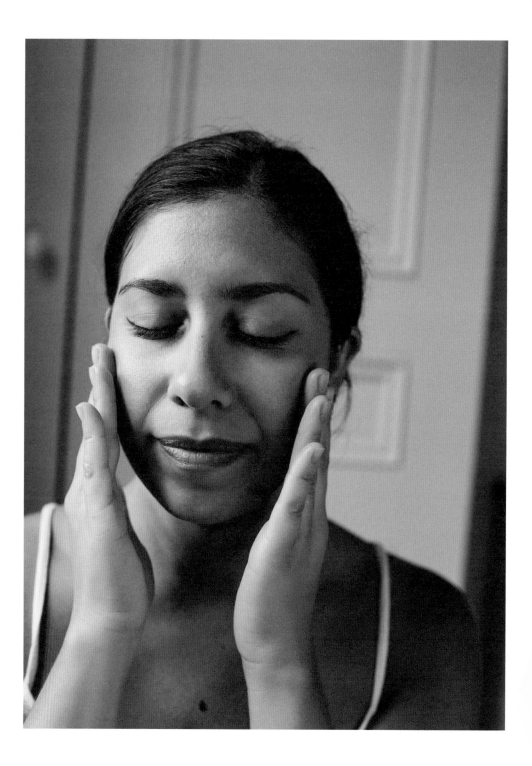

skincare

When you start making your own products you inevitably start learning more about yourself. Let's take skincare: before going zero waste and making my own products I did not know anything about my skin type. I would randomly buy products, and my decision was primarily based on how attractive I felt the packaging was. I did not really pay attention to the materials used to manufacture that packaging and the ingredients inside the product. When I decided to live more zero waste and started making my own products, not only did I pay a lot of attention to packaging materials, but I also really started to learn more about each ingredient in relation to my skin type.

Logically the next question is: how do you know what skin type you have? There are four main skin types: oily, dry, combination and normal. To find out which one you are, look at your skin when you have just woken up and have no make-up on. If you notice your skin has a shiny and oily appearance, specifically on the forehead, and you notice some breakouts (acne and dark spots), then you very likely have oily skin. If your skin tends to feel dry and tight with no breakouts, you have dry skin. If it feels tight but you sometimes feel oiliness or tendency to breakout, then you most likely have combination skin. If you don't notice any oiliness or dryness, then you have normal skin. To help simplify the process of understanding your skin type and skin concern, I have created the chart, overleaf.

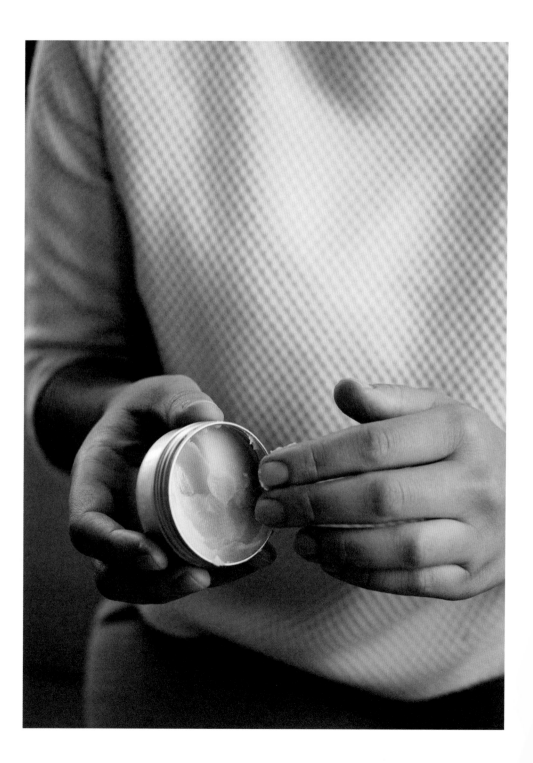

Skin appearance	Result
Shiny, breakouts	Oily skin
Tight, dry, no oily spots or breakouts	Dry skin
Tight, dry with some oily spots and breakouts	Combination skin
No tightness, no dryness, no breakouts	Normal skin

Next, you should identify any skin concerns. For example, you might have rosacea or eczema. If your skin is mature you might have more wrinkles and dark spots. If, on top of the above, your skin is very sensitive, you should really take a lot of care and attention. In fact, this is a simplified way of looking at your skin, and I am not a dermatologist. If you have severe skin concerns – such as rosacea, eczema or severe acne – I highly recommend that you consult a specialist dermatologist before making any skincare decisions.

minimalist skincare routine

Before you start on your first skincare project I want to walk you through all the steps I take and products I use in my minimalist skincare routine, to show you how simple I keep it and what ingredients I normally avoid. This will give you a good overview of how you can incorporate the products in this section into your routine.

The first project involves oil cleansing, a method that works based on the concept that oil dissolves oil. I like to oil cleanse at the end of the day before going to bed to remove any impurities and make-up.

Just after this I also enjoy applying a facial cream. Using your own handmade cream is really such an empowering thing to do, because you get to choose which ingredients to put on your skin. Later in this section you will also learn how to make a rich and hydrating facial cream that is customized according to your needs.

serums

Difficulty level: Beginner
Recipe makes: 30g (1oz)
Shelf life: 6 months

The idea of adding oil to your skin may not sound right – perhaps you think it will clog your pores. Instead, oil cleansing works based on the idea that oil can dissolve oil, so it is a very effective cleansing medium that will not dry your skin. Simply applying a few drops of oil onto your skin will dissolve the sebum on your skin and replace it with new and pure natural oil. I have always struggled with acne and oily skin, but since adopting oil cleansing as part of my routine my skin has improved so much. Oil cleansing is suitable for any skin type – you just need to find the oil that is suited to your skin type by understanding each oil's comedogenic rating. The comedogenic rating determines the likelihood, on a scale from 0 to 5, that an oil will clog your pores – see the chart on pages 62–64.

You can use just one kind of oil, or experiment by mixing different oils in a serum – the way you mix the oils will largely depend on the kind of cleanser you want to make. If you want a cleansing serum, which mainly functions to eliminate dirt, impurities and make-up, I recommend adding some castor oil to your blend. Castor oil is 0 on the comedogenic scale, which means it will not clog your pores; it is thick and viscous and will remove dirt and toxins. You should not use too much of it as it might dry the skin. For a more hydrating serum, which locks in moisture, I highly recommend skipping the castor oil and using a blend of oils that can prevent water loss while keeping your skin light and not greasy. Finally, if you wish to make your serum easier to rinse off, you can include polyglyceryl-4 oleate

– an emulsifier that allows oil and water to mix and so transforms the oil into a milky lotion when in contact with water. You should use only high quality oils – see pages 20–21 for buying advice. Here are some of my favourite serum recipes, with alternative ingredients for different skin types and the method of application for each. Feel free to consult the oil charts on pages 62–64 and make your own version, depending on which oils are easier to source for you.

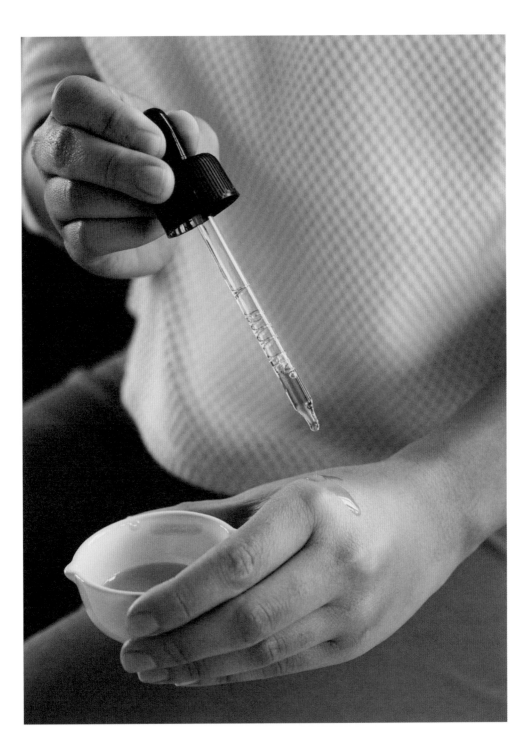

ingredients

Rinse-off cleanser base (optional)

Ingredient name	Comedogenic rating	%	Grams (g)	Ounces (oz)
Oil or oil mix of your choice	2	90.0%	27.00	0.95
Polyglyceryl-4 Oleate	2	10.0%	3.00	0.11
Total ingredients		**100.0%**	**30**	**1.06**

Cleansing and make-up remover serum (oily skin)

Ingredient name	Notes	Comedogenic rating	%	Grams (g)	Ounces (oz)
Grapeseed oil	High in linoleic acid, mild astringent, softens the skin	1	60.0%	18.00	0.63
Hemp seed oil	High in linoleic acid, a dry oil that is emollient but does not clog pores	0	34.0%	10.20	0.36
Castor oil	High in ricinoleic acid, slow absorption and ability to pull out dirt and toxins clearing the skin	0	5.5%	1.65	0.06
Vitamin E oil	Optional if not included in the hemp seed and grapeseed oil; extends the shelf life of grapeseed and hemp seed oil	2	0.5%	0.15	0.01
Total ingredients			**100.0%**	**30**	**1.06**

Cleansing and make-up remover serum (dry or mature skin)

Ingredient name	Notes	Comedogenic rating	%	Grams (g)	Ounces (oz)
Sweet almond oil	High in oleic acid, a very light and emollient oil great for sensitive skin	2	48.0%	14.40	0.51
Avocado oil	High in oleic acid, a very rich and nourishing oil	2	48.0%	14.40	0.51
Castor oil	High in ricinoleic acid, slow absorption and ability to pull out dirt and toxins clearing the skin	0	4.0%	1.20	0.04
Total ingredients			**100.0%**	**30**	**1.06**

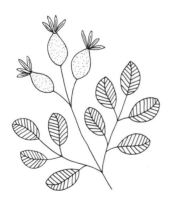

Light, seal-in moisture serum (oily/acne prone skin)

Ingredient name	Notes	Comedogenic rating	%	Grams (g)	Ounces (oz)
Argan oil	High in oleic acid	0	55.0%	16.50	0.58
Hemp seed oil	High in linoleic acid	0	38.5%	11.55	0.40
Rosehip oil	High in oleic acid, omega 3, vitamin A (beta carotene) and vitamin E, repairs damaged skin tissue	1	5.0%	1.50	0.05
Tamanu oil	Anti-inflammatory against acne and eczema	2	0.5%	0.15	0.01
Helichrysum essential oil	Optional for acne prone skin and healing acne scars	N/A	0.5%	0.15	0.01
Vitamin E oil	Optional if not included in the hemp seed; extends the shelf life of hemp seed oil	2	0.5%	0.15	0.01
Total ingredients			**100.0%**	**30**	**1.06**

Light, seal-in moisture serum (normal/combination/dry/mature skin)

Notes	Ingredient name	Comedogenic rating	%	Grams (g)	Ounces (oz)
Jojoba	Natural temporary occlusive (seals in moisture)	2	48.0%	14.40	0.51
Evening primrose oil	High in linoleic acid	2	48.0%	14.40	0.51
Sea buckthorn CO_2 extract	Rich in vitamin A (beta carotene), regenerates skin cells	1	3.5%	1.05	0.04
Vitamin E oil	Optional if not included in the evening primrose oil; extends the shelf life of evening primrose oil	2	0.5%	0.15	0.01
Total ingredients			**100.0%**	**30**	**1.06**

equipment

- High precision scales
- Bowl
- Teaspoon
- Stainless steel saucepan (optional)
- 30g (1oz) glass bottle with pipette
- Optional: a mini plastic funnel of about 4 x 3cm (1½ x 1in)

safety notes

- Make sure the hot face towel in used to remove the cleanser (see right) is not too hot.
- Avoid using castor oil during pregnancy as it may cause contractions.

instructions

1. If you are making a serum containing just oils and vitamin E, simply add all the ingredients together into a bowl, mix well with a teaspoon or spatula, and transfer the mixture into a glass bottle with the help of a small funnel or using a teaspoon. Alternatively, you could also add the ingredients straight into the glass bottle with the help of a small funnel, and shake well to incorporate the ingredients.

2. Instead, if you wish to create a cleanser with the addition of Polyglyceryl-4 Oleate, add the ingredients in a heat-safe bowl to be heated in a bain-marie (see page 29) to 70°C (158°F), and then mix until cooled down.

3. Pour the mixture into the glass bottle with the help of a mini funnel or a teaspoon or using the pipette of the glass bottle.

how to use the serums and cleansers

Apply a few drops of the cleanser into the palm of your hand and start massaging your face gently. To remove make-up from your eyes, massage really gently making sure to keep your eye closed at all times. Finally, place a face cloth under hot (not burning) water, rinse off any excess cleanser and place it on your face. The steam will completely dissolve any leftover oil and dirt and you will be left with incredibly soft and purified skin.

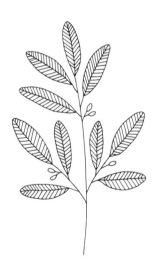

facial cream

Difficulty level: Advanced
Recipe makes: 30g (1oz)
Shelf life: 6 months

When approaching the world of zero-waste living there is a difficult decision to make about a particular product: face cream. Here is why: most zero-waste products are solid and water-free because this reduces or eliminates the need for any packaging. However, when it comes to creams – especially face creams – it's tricky to find one that does not come packaged in single-use plastic because for a good cream to be very effective, but also light and quick to absorb, water must be introduced into the formula. Since water and oils naturally do not mix well together you will need to add an emulsifier, which will allow oils and water to bind into a cream. Making a cream from scratch allows you to pick every single ingredient depending on your skin type. Not only can you choose exactly what oils to include but you can also customize the 'water' part of the recipe. For example, you could use aloe vera juice or hydrolates, which are infused flower waters that are a by-product of essential oil distillation – examples are rose water or chamomile hydrosol. This means that the recipe formulation will be a little bit more complicated than just melting a few butters together. However, the result will be incredible and, trust me, you will never go back to store-bought creams!

The only problem you might encounter when trying to make your own cream from scratch is that the recipes available on the internet look so incredibly complex. For simplification here is a base formula, so you understand how the ingredients interact with each other. By understanding how the structure of a cream works, you will no longer feel scared (at least I know I don't anymore!) whenever you want to try to make a more complex and customized cream. The recipe is divided into two different parts – the water part and the oil part – and the cream is prepared in three separate phases: the heated water phase, the heated oil phase and the cool down phase, which determine the way you should prepare the ingredients.

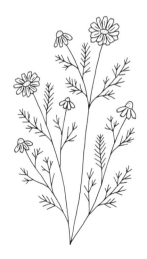

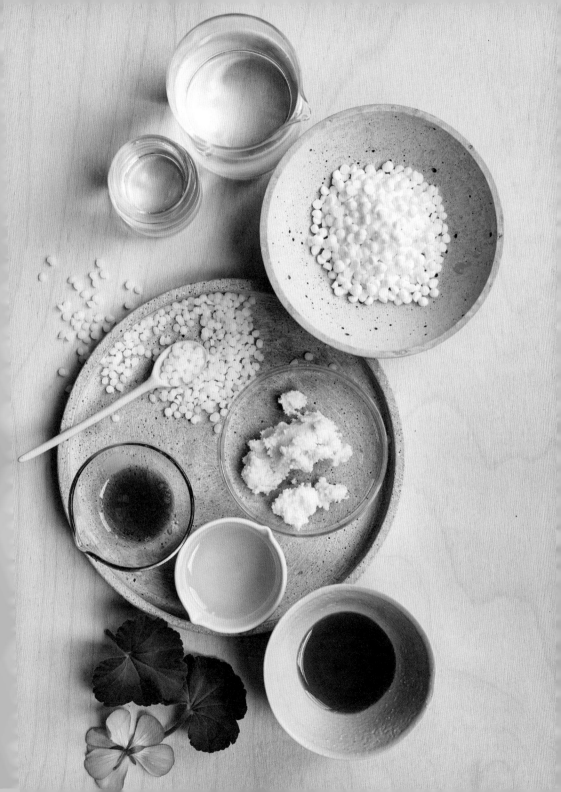

water part

Water makes the biggest bulk of a creams recipe, at around 60–80% of the total recipe. The less water you use, the thicker the cream will be and vice versa. In this recipe the water is at 75% so it will make up the bulk of the recipe – this will give a thin yet rich cream consistency. Use distilled water as opposed to tap water.

oil part

The oil part of a basic cream is generally made up of:
- Oils and/or butters (to nourish and soften the skin).
- Emulsifying wax (allows the oils to mix with the water part).
- Co-emulsifier (increases the stability of the cream so oil and water don't separate).
- Preservative (mandatory to preserve the cream).
- Fragrance (optional, to scent the cream).

heated and cool down phases

The ingredients in both the water and the oil part will need to be heated to 70°C (158°F) in the heating phases. In fact, both phases need to be at the same temperature when mixed together. During the heating phase any solid ingredients will also gently melt down until fully liquid and ready to incorporate. When heating the water ingredients some will actually evaporate and you can compensate this loss by adding the lost amount after you take the beaker off the heat. However, I do not believe this is strictly necessary if you are making a small batch because the loss will be really small. The heating phase will reach quite a high temperature and not all the ingredients

are suitable for this because they could lose some of their precious nutrients and properties in the process. These thermolabile ingredients will be added only at the very last step during the cool down phase, below 45°C (113°F). To further simplify and distinguish each phase from each other, formulators often use letters next to each phase (A, B, C, D, etc).

emulsification

Emulsification refers to the stage when the water is added to the oils, and these mix together to form a cream. To achieve a complete and stable emulsification it is important to whisk using an electric mini whisk or a stick blender. Depending on the ingredients and ratios used, some creams will thicken straight away, while others might need to rest for a few minutes before fully thickening up.

pH

As long as the ingredients used are pH balanced, you should not need to test or adjust the pH of your cream – adjusting the pH of a cream is an advanced technique not covered in this book.

ingredients

base cream recipe

Phase	Ingredient name	Structure	%	Grams (g)	Ounces (oz)
Heated water phase (A)	Distilled water	Water	71.7%	21.51	0.76
Heated oil phase (B)	Jojoba	Oil	20.0%	6.00	0.21
	Olivem 1000	Emulsifier	5.0%	1.50	0.05
	Cetyl alcohol	Co-emulsifier	2.0%	0.60	0.02
Cool down phase (C)	Preservative	Preservative	0.8%	0.24	0.01
	Essential oil	Fragrance	0.5%	0.15	0.01
	Total ingredients		**100.0%**	**30**	**1.06**

equipment
- Tight-fitting rubber gloves (optional)
- Stainless steel saucepan
- High precision scales
- 3 heat-safe beakers
- Thermometer
- Electric mini whisk or stick blender
- Teaspoon or spatula
- 30g (1oz) wide-mouthed aluminium or glass jar with lid, or upcycled plastic jar

safety notes
Sterilize any tool you will be using with surgical spirit (rubbing alcohol).

Wash your hands well and work in a clean area. If you wish you can wear a pair of clean, tight-fitting rubber gloves.

The high amount of water in increases the risk of bacteria forming so it is very important not to use tap water in facial creams.

Since germs and bacteria can form in the presence of water, you must preserve this cream with a broad-spectrum preservative.

Using nutrient-rich, water-soluble ingredients, such as floral hydrosol or aloe vera juice, will result in a microbially less stable cream. As a consequence, if you make any changes to the water portion of the cream you might need to increase the usage rate of your preservative.

Certain oils have a short shelf life of about six months, so I recommend adding vitamin E to improve their stability.

Depending on which preservative you decide to use, it is your responsibility to test the efficacy of your preservative system. You can do so by checking with your supplier and contacting a certified cosmetic chemist to assist you in the assessment of the safety of your formulation.

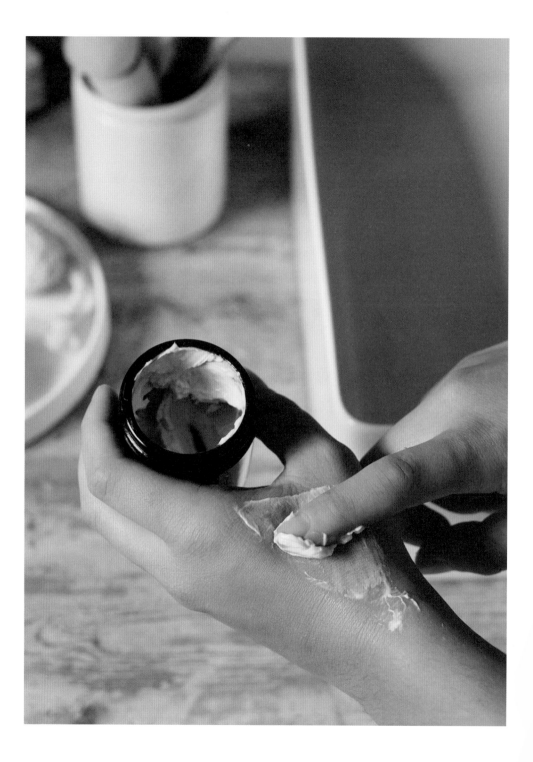

instructions

1. Make a bain-marie as described on page 29. In the meantime, weigh the ingredients into three separate heat-safe beakers, one for each phase as described on page 68.

2. When the water has started simmering, place the heated water phase ingredients and the heated oil phase ingredients into the saucepan within their beakers.

3. Allow to simmer until all the solid heated oil ingredients have melted completely. For 30g (1oz) of cream, and depending on the ingredients you are using, it should take around 10 minutes.

4. Turn off the heat, remove the two beakers from the water bath and check that the contents of both beakers have reached 70°C (158°F). If so, pour the contents of the water beaker into the oil beaker.

5. Blend with a mini whisk or a stick blender until you start seeing the first stage of emulsification: the oils and the water will bind together creating a white, milk-consistency cream.

6. Measure the temperature of the cream; when the mixture has cooled down to below 45°C (113°F), add the cool down phase ingredients – the preservative and the optional essential oils – and mix with a clean teaspoon or spatula. During this cool down phase, you will notice that the cream will start thickening up. If the mixture is still quite runny, blend for a few more seconds until you obtain a soft and fluffy cream. If the cream is not thickening up and remains runny, don't worry too much – depending on the emulsifier you used, it might thicken up once it's completely cooled down.

7. Transfer the cream into a clean and sterilized jar or tin. Sterilize by spraying the jar or tin with rubbing alcohol and wiping dry with a clean cloth/paper towel. Allow the cream to cool down before closing the lid to avoid condensation, which could cause water droplets to contaminate the cream.

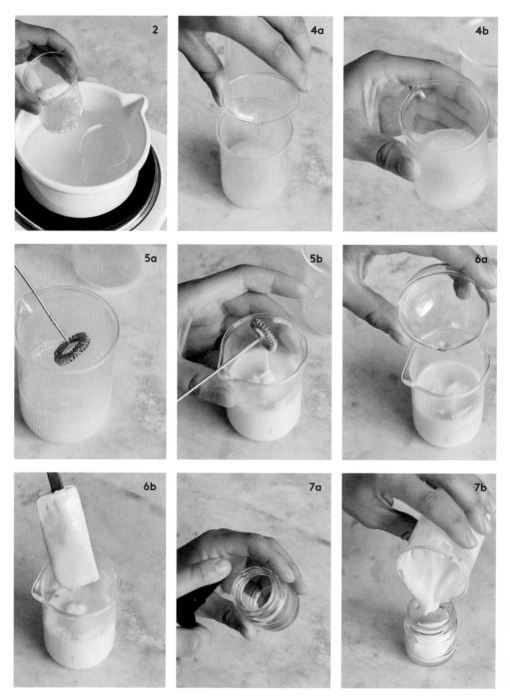

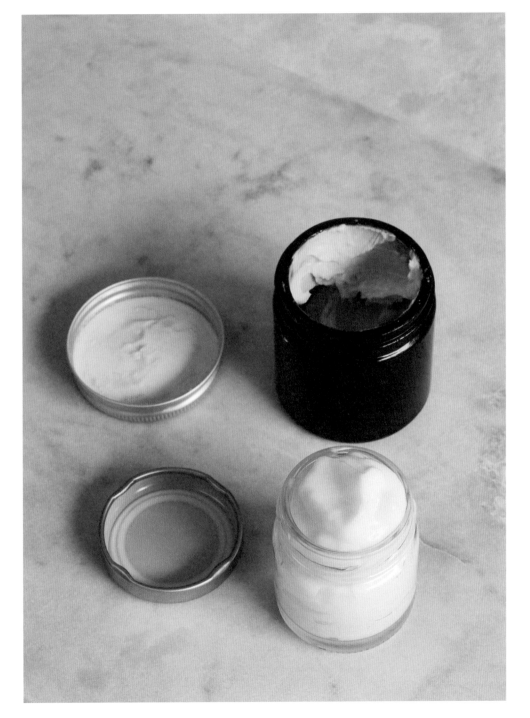

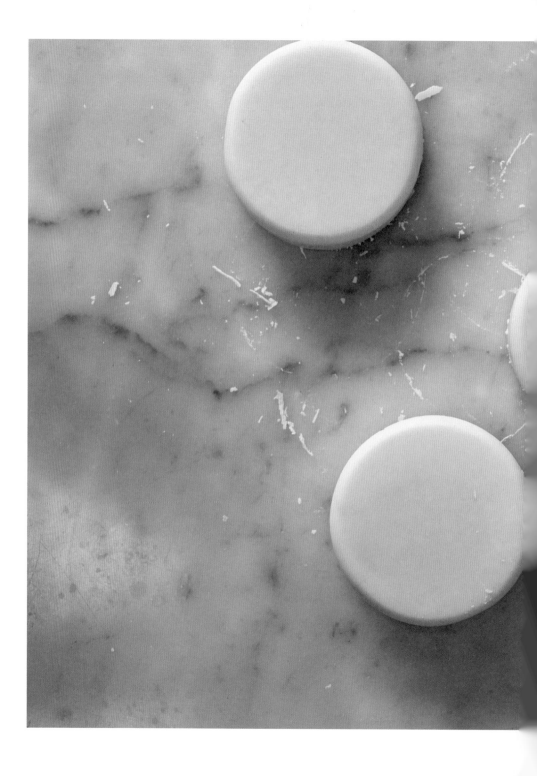

soap

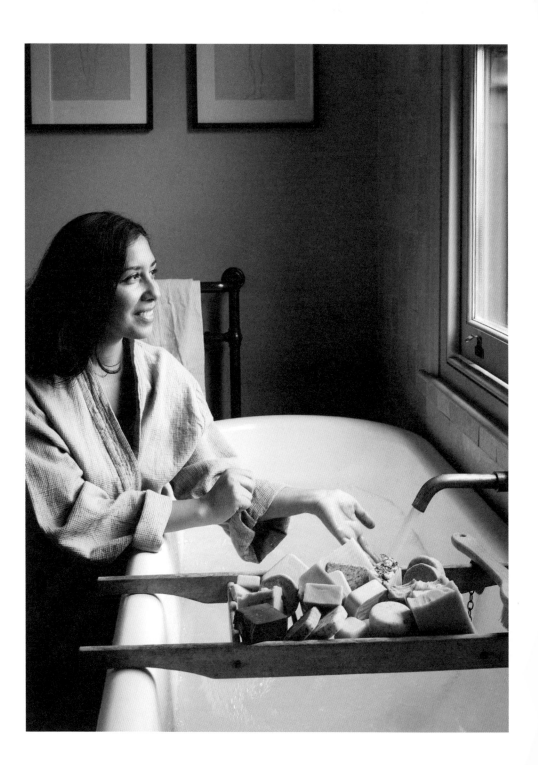

soap

What truly fascinates me is that if two soap makers make the same recipe, they will likely end up with two very different soaps – soap is the outcome of a very precise science but it can sometimes be very unpredictable. Not only the ingredients, but also apparently small things like the temperature of the room you are in and even the speed at which you are soaping can all affect the final outcome.

So, what is soap? It is the result of a reaction that happens when the fats contained in oils/butters come into contact with an alkaline (high pH) solution, called sodium hydroxide (NaoH). Sodium hydroxide (also called caustic soda or lye) first needs to be dissolved into a liquid, which is normally water but could also be any other liquid (milk, tea, wine...). When mixed it becomes a lye solution, which heats up and can reach up to 93°C (200°F). Since sodium hydroxide is a caustic ingredient, **you must be very careful when making soap and wear all the protective equipment (see pages 86–87).** Mixing the lye solution and the oils results in the soap thickening up until it reaches a solid state.

There are different methods to make soap. In this book we will explore the cold-process method, which is one of the most popular for a very good reason: it relies only on a natural saponification process with no added heat other than the heat that is naturally created during the saponification reaction. This also helps preserve the essential qualities of the ingredients used, which would be destroyed if the mixture was cooked. The cold-process method requires about four to six weeks before the soap can be used – when it is first made your soap will still be caustic and needs to cure. This means that all the liquid that you mixed with the sodium hydroxide needs to evaporate for the soap to become mild and gentle on the skin. Soap making is truly a labour of love and has taught me how to become patient and appreciate the slower movement of natural things! The anticipation behind waiting for a soap to become usable is priceless and I really hope you will be able to experience it too.

overview of the soap-making process

Your chosen oils and/or butters need to be melted. The lye solution is prepared by adding the sodium hydroxide to the water (**never** the opposite). This lye solution, which is heated to around 43°C (110°F) (this is dependent on the type of soap you are making, see page 82), is then added into the oils (not the opposite) you have chosen to use in your soap. At this point you need to blend the two elements, and this is normally done with a stick blender to speed up the process (using a spoon would take hours!). Within a matter of seconds, the mixture will start to thicken until it reaches a stage called 'trace' (see page 82), which has the consistency of a light, smooth custard. This is normally the step where you will add any extras such as essential oils. Even if the soap-making reaction is still happening, it will not be as strong as when you first added the lye solution to the oils so any precious properties contained in the essential oils will be preserved.

The more you stick blend, the harder the batter will become, but you don't want it to become too thick – it needs to be smooth and pourable. Once the mixture thickens up, there is no turning back; the soap will become harder and harder until it reaches a solid state. While the soap batter is still light and pourable it is poured into a flexible mould, which is usually silicone or a wooden mould with a paper lining. The soap is then usually insulated and left to harden for 24 hours. The following day you are ready to unmould the soap and unveil your beautiful creation. I get chills even just thinking about this! Trust me when I say this is one of the best moments of the soap-making process.

You can make soap with virtually any fat, from olive oil to beef tallow. Each oil will give unique characteristics to your soap, such as fluffy lather and hardness. You can decide which attributes you want your soap to have by looking at each oil's profile in the chart on page 90.

You can colour and scent your soaps naturally or with synthetic colours and fragrances, but in this book I explore the art of making soap with vegetable fats, botanical colours and essential oils. I also do not use any palm oil in my soap recipes, because it is quite a controversial ingredient that often comes from an unsustainable supply chain.

In each recipe you can use up to 3% of the total oils – do not exceed this amount. As long as you stick to the proportions, you can use a blend of different essential oils – just make sure to research their properties, allergens and possible contraindications.

how to make lye solution

Keep your gloves and goggles on, and wear your mask/respirator if you have one, or a scarf over your nose and mouth. To prepare the lye solution, add the sodium hydroxide to the water and stir well with a stainless steel tablespoon to dissolve it fully, make sure not to cause splashes. Put the lye solution in a safe spot away from pets and children until it cools down to 43°C (110°F). Monitor the temperature using a thermometer.

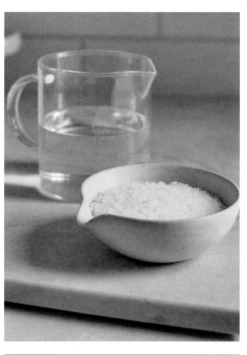
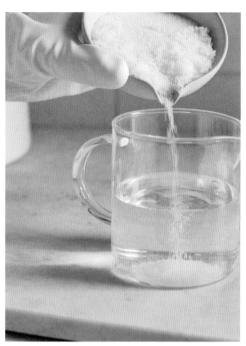
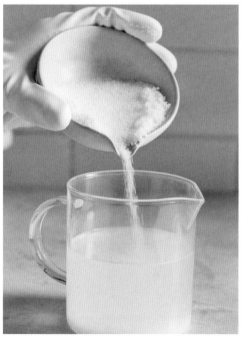
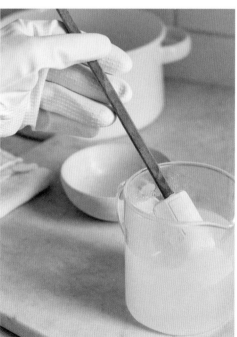

soap-making oils chart

Most of the oils have between a one- to two- years shelf life. See notes for those with a short shelf life. Please note these are indicative ranges, not rules set in stone.

Ingredient	Lather	Hardness (0-4)	Usage rate	Notes
Apricot kernel oil	Conditioning	0	5–15%	Best for dry and sensitive skin, will soften the soap
Avocado oil	Conditioning, creamy	1	5–15%	Best for dry skin, leaves a slightly greasy feel
Babassu oil	Cleansing, fluffy	4	5–33%	Best for lather and hardness. Can be drying
Canola oil	Conditioning, creamy and low lather	0	10–20%	Usually used as a partial substitute for the more expensive olive oil
Castor oil	conditioning and fluffy	0	3–20%	Used for large, conditioning lather but will soften the soap
Cocoa butter	Conditioning, creamy	4	5–10%	Used for hardness, too much can make the soap gummy (10%) or brittle (>10%). Unrefined kind can carry the smell through
Coconut oil	Cleansing and fluffy	4	5–33%	Best for lather and hardness. Can be drying. Unrefined kind can carry the smell through
Grapeseed oil	Conditioning, low lather	0	3–10%	Best for conditioning in low amounts. Makes soap soft and has short shelf life
Hemp seed oil	Conditioning, low lather	0	3–10%	Best for conditioning in low amounts. Makes soap soft and has short shelf life
Kokum butter	Conditioning, low lather	4	5–10%	Good alternative to cocoa butter, makes the soap harder
Jojoba oil	Conditioning, low lather	0	3–10%	Best for extra conditioning in low amounts. Makes soap soft and can reduce the lather. It is also expensive
Mango butter	Conditioning, low lather	3	5–15%	Used for hardness, more expensive than cocoa butter
Neem oil	Conditioning, low lather	2	3–5%	Conditioning, often used for pet soaps or sensitive skin

Ingredient	Lather	Hardness (0-4)	Usage rate	Notes
Olive oil	Conditioning and creamy	0*	up to 100%	Best for dry and sensitive skin. It will harden over time. Really low lather
Rice bran oil	Silky and conditioning	2	5–20%	Best for dry skin, contributes to hardness. Can be used as a partial substitute for the more expensive olive oil
Rapeseed oil	Silky and conditioning	0	5–15%	Best for dry skin, too much will soften the soap. Often referred to as canola oil, which is a is a kind of rapeseed oil usually used in food
Shea butter	Conditioning and creamy	3	5–15%	Best for dry skin, contributes to hardness. Too much (>15%) inhibits lather. Unrefined kind carries the smell through when over 10%
Sweet almond oil	Conditioning	0	5-15%	Used for hardness, too much (>10%) will soften the soap
Sunflower oil	Silky and conditioning	0	5–20%	Best for adding conditioning and silkiness to the lather. The high oleic kind is prone to rancidity

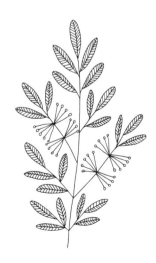

trace

Trace is a phase in soap making that appears after you have combined the lye solution with the water and stick blended a little – at this point, if you let the soap batter drip across its own surface it will leave a trail behind. This is a very crucial part of the soap-making process as from this stage there is no turning back: the soap will start to thicken up until solid.

light trace: this stage happens after a few seconds of first stick blending the lye solution into the soap – it has a similar consistency to a really runny lotion. This is the time to add any essential oils and additives into your soap.

medium trace: this is generally achieved after you have stick blended for a few more seconds after you have reached a light trace. This stage has the consistency of a light custard and is normally when you want to pour the soap into the mould.

thick trace: at this stage the soap becomes much thicker and harder to pour and has a consistency similar to mayonnaise. If you have poured at this stage, make sure to tap the mould really well otherwise you will end up with unaesthetic air pockets within your soap.

After these stages the soap will start to thicken even more until it no longer becomes pourable, and it fully solidifies into soap. A sudden thickening of the soap is called 'trace acceleration' and can happen with certain essential oils and fragrances, heavy additives like clays and powders, or recipes that contain a lot of butters and heavy oils such as castor oil.

temperature

The temperature you choose to soap at will depend on the type of recipe. A standard soaping temperature is 43°C (110°F), but you can also choose to soap at a higher temperature of 49°C (120°F). In more advanced recipes that include heat-sensitive ingredients containing milk or sugars, you normally soap at much lower temperatures of 26°C (80°F) to 32°C (90°F).

It is okay if the temperature is not exactly as the above. However, whatever temperature you choose, you need to be sure that the oils and the lye solution are not more than 6°C (10°F) degrees apart from each other.

superfatting soap

Saponification is the chemical reaction in which the fats and oils react with the lye to form soap. Each oil has a unique saponification value (SAP), which determines the amount of sodium hydroxide required to fully saponify the given amount of fat (in our case, oil) in a recipe. For example, the SAP value of olive oil is 0.135, meaning you need 0.13g of sodium hydroxide to transform 1 gram of olive oil into soap. Don't worry, you won't need to calculate the amount of sodium hydroxide required – there are specific softwares that can do that for you. One of the best can be found at SoapCalc.net and is completely free (see page 85). Once you know the SAP value you can then decide to discount (reduce) the amount of sodium hydroxide required, which will leave more oil in the soap, making it gentler to the skin. This process is also called 'superfatting' because you are leaving some oils in the soap unsaponified making the soap 'fatter'. A standard superfat amount used by most soap makers is 5% – this is a safe amount that does not make your soap too soft or go rancid faster. However, you can also decide to saponify oils at 6%, 7%, 10%, 15% or 20%. Coconut oil has a long shelf life of about two years – it's a hard, cleansing oil – so this is one of the very few oils you can safely superfat up to 20%, to obtain an excellent fluffy body soap.

water and water discounts

Water, or another chosen liquid, is primarily needed to dissolve the sodium hydroxide to create the lye solution. If your tap water is good enough to drink, you should not have any problems making soap with it. That being said, if you are planning to sell your soap you might consider using distilled or deionized water. It is important to learn how to use water in soap making because it determines the strength of your lye solution. A more concentrated lye solution is ideal for soap recipes such as the 100% olive oil soap, where the oil will take longer to reach trace, because this will speed up the trace. A weaker lye solution will be more beneficial in a 100% coconut oil recipe, as this will slow down the trace time.

The most common ratio of sodium hydroxide to water is called full water, which is a 25% lye solution: 25% sodium hydroxide; 75% water. The next is a moderate water discount, which normally uses 33% sodium hydroxide and 67% water. A strong water discount of 40% sodium hydroxide and 60% water can be applied for different reasons. The maximum water discount you can apply is 50% sodium hydroxide and 50% water. Sodium hydroxide cannot dissolve itself into a liquid smaller than its own weight, so if you use less than 50% water you will have a dangerously lye-heavy soap.

lye solution checklist

- Sodium hydroxide cannot dissolve itself into an amount of liquid smaller than its own weight.

- The amount of water in a soap recipe does not change depending on which oils you are using, but it determines the strength or weakness of the lye solution.

- You can substitute other liquids for water – but because the temperature will rise when the lye is added to the liquid, some liquids (such as milk) will require more advanced handling.

- More water in your soap can make the soap overheat and pass through a phase called 'gel'. Gel phase is perfect if you want any colours in your soap to pop out more.

- The water added to your soap will need to evaporate out eventually. The more water you add, the slower your soap will trace, and the slower it will take to cure and harden.

- Adding some sodium lactate to the cooled down lye solution before it's poured into the oils can help produce a harder and longer lasting bar or soap with a smoother finish. The recommended usage rate is about 5g (0.18oz) or 1 teaspoon for every 450g (16oz) of soap.

- When you add the sodium hydroxide to the water be sure to stir it very gently (so not to cause any splashes) but straight away, without waiting, otherwise it will start to solidify and will create a few hard to dissolve clumps.

25% lye solution

33% lye solution

40% lye solution

50% lye solution

key
The light grey is water
The dark grey is sodium hydroxide

gel phase

Gel phase occurs during the heating phase of the saponification process. It is called gel because it makes the soap look exactly like gel – quite translucent – and the result is that any colours you put in your soap will pop out more.

using online calculators

Soap Calc is a free online tool where you can just type in details of your formulation to obtain a calculation of the exact quantity of each ingredient that will be required to achieve the desired result. You can access it at soapcalc.net/calc/SoapCalcWP.asp and for instruction on how to use the software visit soapcalc.net/info/helptext.asp.

substitutions

If you want to change up the oils in any recipe, you will need to re-run the whole recipe through a lye calculator again. This is because each oil requires a very specific amount of sodium hydroxide to become soap (see Superfatting Soap on pages 83).

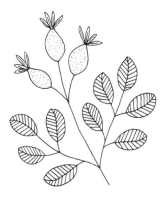

soap safety measures

Before diving into the making of your first soap, it is **very** important that you familiarize yourself with essential safety measures. As mentioned previously, sodium hydroxide is a very caustic material, which heats up and reaches very high temperatures when in contact with a liquid. If you get a splash of sodium hydroxide on your skin it can burn down tissues very easily. I don't mean to scare you (or maybe just a little) but it is incredibly important that you follow the safety measures diligently. Handling lye will become just like learning how to drive: if you drive without care and attention it is dangerous but if you follow the safety measures, like wearing a seat belt and respecting the speed limit, then you will be safe. Naturally you might be thinking: can you make soap without lye? The answer is that soap does not exist without lye – it is formed by the very reaction between an oil and the sodium hydroxide. Although you could use a ready 'melt and pour' soap base, this is an artificial soap base that is normally sold in plastic and will not help you on your zero-waste journey.

soap-making safety checklist

- **protect your eyes** by always wearing a pair of safety goggles when handling lye and raw soap, even if you wear glasses.

- **protect your hands and body** by wearing a pair of reusable rubber gloves, and if possible, long sleeves and long trousers.

- **make sure your area is free from children or pets** and never leave lye solution unattended. Never make soap with little ones around and make sure any lye or sodium hydroxide is clearly labelled and stored out of reach.

- **soap in a well-ventilated area and wear a mask or respirator** when you are adding the lye to the water. The heat reaction will produce a few fumes that you don't want to breathe in. If you don't have a mask you can use a scarf or hold your breath.

- **always, always add the sodium hydroxide to the water and never the opposite** – if you do the opposite, the reaction will be too strong and the solution could 'erupt' from its container. If I forget I play this song in my head: **if you add the water to the lye, you will die. Add the lye to the water to make it proper!** Yes, it is really dramatic but it is the only way I remembered at the beginning!

- **if you get lye on you, immediately wash off with cold running water** and seek medical help. If you ingest any lye, absolutely do not induce vomiting because this will cause the lye to come back up in your throat and can burn it.

- **use the correct containers** – you will need heat-safe glass, stainless steel or very heavy-duty plastic bowls that can withstand temperatures up to 93°C (200°F). Never use aluminium bowls for soap making, as this metal can react with the sodium hydroxide.

- **avoid wooden utensils** as they can be damaged by the sodium hydroxide over time. Silicone works well for moulds and spatulas; avoid plastic or metal moulds – you need a flexible material to get the soap out of the mould after it has been poured.

- **have dedicated soap making tools** – any tools that you use for soap-making should never be used afterwards for food purposes.

dealing with soda ash

Soda ash is a white coating that commonly forms when air comes in contact with unreacted sodium hydroxide – it is completely harmless but could ruin the soap's final aesthetic. In general, this happens in soaps that either have not been insulated properly whilst in the mould, contain a lot of water, or have been poured when the batter was too thin. If you are making a colourful soap pay extra attention to soda ash, because if it forms it will be very noticeable. One way to avoid it forming is to spray the poured soap with 99.9% isopropyl alcohol. Pouring the soap when it's not too liquid and insulating the soap with a piece of cardboard and a blanket will also help, however you will need to be careful not to over-blend the soap, which would result in a thick and hard-to-pour mixture. If you do get soda ash, you can try to remove it from the unmoulded soap using a hand-held steamer for a few seconds, by rubbing it off with a piece of wet cloth, or by cutting off the affected area completely.

how to choose the oil quality and kind

When purchasing oil, keep in mind that you can use any quality or type, but this will impact the final result.In general, unrefined oils or butters contain more fats and nutrients than their refined counterparts. However, they are also more prone to rancidity and may produce a strong scent or colour in the final soap.

For example, olive oil is available in a pure olive oil, extra virgin olive oil or pomace oil. The pure olive oil is normally a mix of refined and unrefined oil and has a pale colour, making it a suitable choice if you are making coloured soaps.

The extra virgin and the pomace oil are both fattier and darker in colour. The difference is extra virgin is much more expensive, while pomace oil is a lower grade olive oil, obtained from the olive pulp after the first press.

Similarly, when choosing between coconut oil, shea butter and cocoa butter, you can use both the refined or unrefined versions, keeping the above in mind.

coconut and olive body soap

Difficulty level: Beginner
Recipe makes: 100g (3.5oz) of soap,
**   about 1–2 soaps depending on the**
**   size of the mould used**
Cure time: 4–6 weeks
Shelf life: 6 months

When I first started soap making I was looking for
a recipe for a soap that could be used both for my
hands and body, so I would be able to replace the
liquid soap and shower gel with one single product.
The key ingredients that will give this result are
olive oil and coconut oil. Olive oil is very high in oleic
acid, so it contributes to making the soap gentle
and to nourishing the skin. Coconut oil provides
hardness and luxurious bubbles, which is exactly
what you need in a body soap! I recommend adding
a blend of lavender and sweet orange essential oil,
which creates a sweet, refreshing, very relaxing and
long-lasting scent.

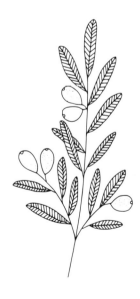

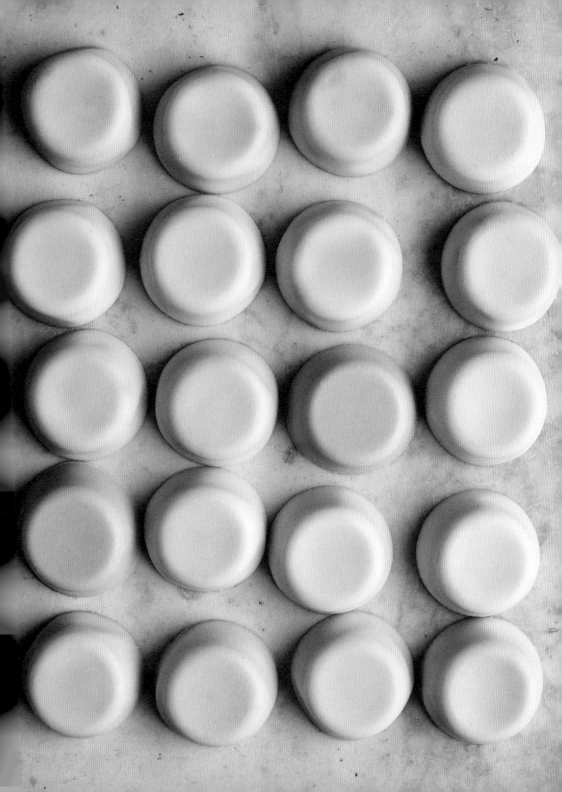

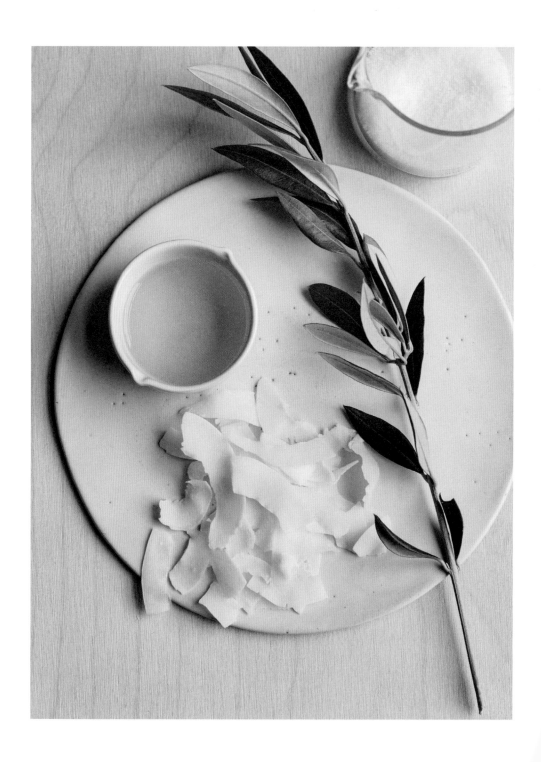

ingredients
lye solution (33% lye concentration, 5% superfat)
- 28.89g (1.02oz) water
- 14.23g (0.50oz) sodium hydroxide

oils
- 70% olive oil: 70g (2.47oz)
- 30% coconut oil: 30g (1oz)
- Optional: 3g (0.10oz) of essential oils (3% of your total oil quantity, which in this case is 100g/3.52oz)
- Optional: 1.10g (0.03oz) of sodium lactate will help increase the hardiness of the soap

recommended soaping temperature
43°C (110°F)

equipment
- Goggles
- Gloves
- High precision scales
- 2 heat-safe glass or stainless steel jugs
- Ceramic or glass bowl
- Mask/respirator or scarf
- Stainless steel tablespoon
- Thermometer
- Stainless steel saucepan
- Silicone spatula
- Stick blender
- Moulds

safety notes
For this recipe use up to 3g (0.10oz) of essential oils (3% of the total oils). Do not exceed this amount.

Keep goggles and gloves on at all times when handling lye and raw soap.

Work in a well-ventilated area and keep children and pets away.

Do not weigh the sodium hydroxide in an aluminium container, or in a very light paper or plastic one.

Add the sodium hydroxide to the water and never the opposite.

instructions

1. Wearing goggles and gloves, weigh the sodium hydroxide (see Safety Notes on page 91).

2. Weigh the water in a separate heat-safe glass or stainless steel container.

3. Keep your gloves and goggles on, and wear your mask/respirator if you have one, or a scarf over your nose and mouth. To prepare the lye solution, add the sodium hydroxide to the water and stir well with a stainless steel tablespoon to dissolve it fully; make sure not to cause splashes. Put the lye solution in a safe spot away from pets and children until it cools down to 43°C (110°F). Monitor the temperature using a thermometer.

4. While the lye solution is cooling down, weigh the olive oil and the coconut oil in a heat-safe jug or stainless steel saucepan, and gently melt the coconut oil and heat up the olive oil. You can place the oils in the stainless steel saucepan on very low heat, or melt them using a bain-marie (see page 29), or in the microwave. This should take just a few minutes: monitor the oils and make sure not to overheat them.

5. At this point weigh your essential oils inside a small bowl or beaker, if using, and keep them on the side ready to be used in one of the next steps. Prepare the moulds you want to use for your soaps.

6. Once the olive and coconut oil are both at around 43°C (110°F), add the lye solution (which is also around the same temperature) to the oils and gently stir with a spatula.

7. Stick blend until you reach trace (see page 82). If you want to add the essential oils, do this at a very light trace and stick blend a little bit more until you notice that the soap leaves a light trail when dripped on the batter's surface.

8. Pour the mixture into the moulds and tap to remove any air bubbles. Spray with 99.9% isopropyl alcohol, if preferred, to prevent soda ash.

9. Cover the soap with a piece of cardboard and add a blanket or a pile of fabric to keep the soap warm and insulated as much as possible. Let the soap harden for 24 hours, then unmould and leave to cure on a clean shelf in a dry room for 4–6 weeks before using.

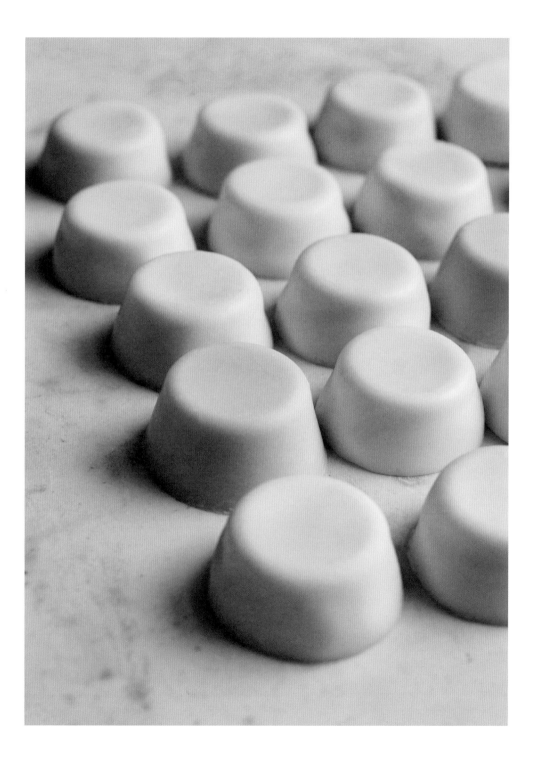

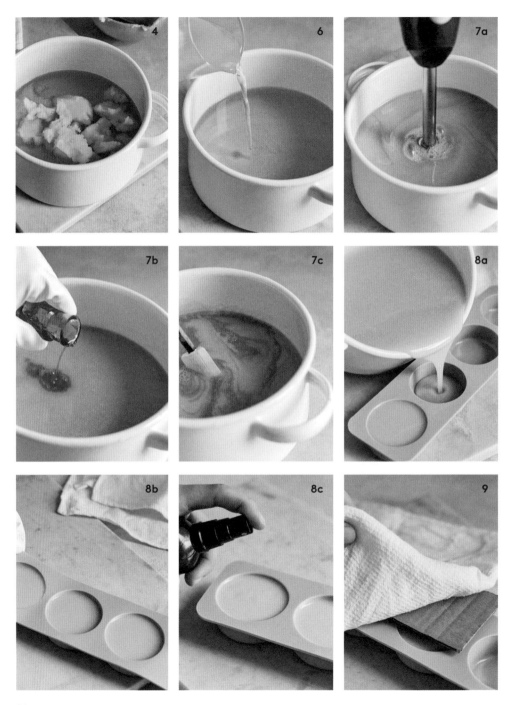

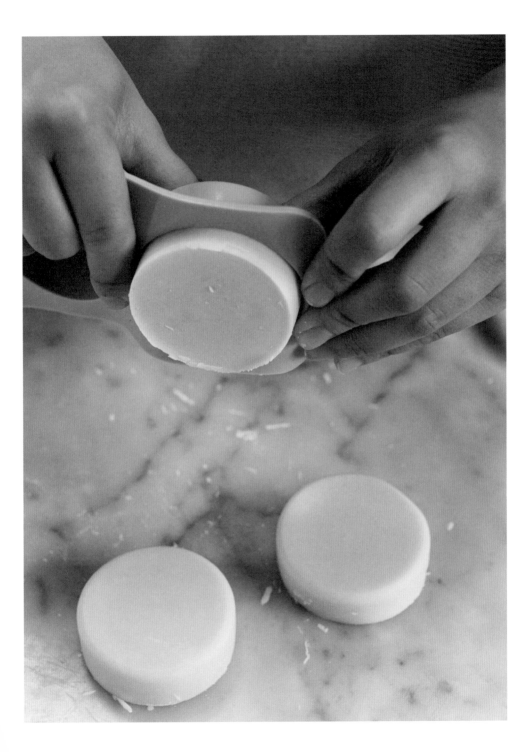

one-oil soaps

I firmly believe that simplicity is at the core of zero-waste living, and in soap making you can obtain some of the most glorious soaps using just one oil. Some of the most flexible oils for this are olive oil and coconut oil; they have a unique fatty acid profile that makes them suitable to use on their own in a soap recipe. Using other oils at 100% in your recipe would not necessarily work – for example, 100% castor oil will make an incredibly soft soap, or 100% cocoa butter will make a brittle soap. The two one-oil soap recipes I have included in this section are Castile Soap on pages 98–99, using 100% olive oil, and Coconut Body or Dishwashing Soap on pages 102–103, using 100% coconut oil.

Olive oil is truly a unique oil because it is incredibly high in oleic acid, which is perfect for very dry and sensitive skin types; it is most recommended if you are looking to make a face or baby soap. Its lather is very low, almost lotion like. It is a soft oil that needs a very long time to cure and harden – although you could use it after the standard cure time of four to six weeks, many soap makers like to leave 100% olive oil soap to cure for six months or even a whole year!

Coconut oil is quite the opposite: it provides bubbles and hardness to your soap bar, but it is also very cleansing so could dry your skin. Soap made with 100% coconut oil would be very suitable as dishwashing, laundry or stain-remover soap. If you want to make 100% coconut oil soap for bodycare, the trick is to discount (reduce) some of the sodium hydroxide in the lye solution to make the soap 'superfatted' (see pages 83) and milder to the skin.

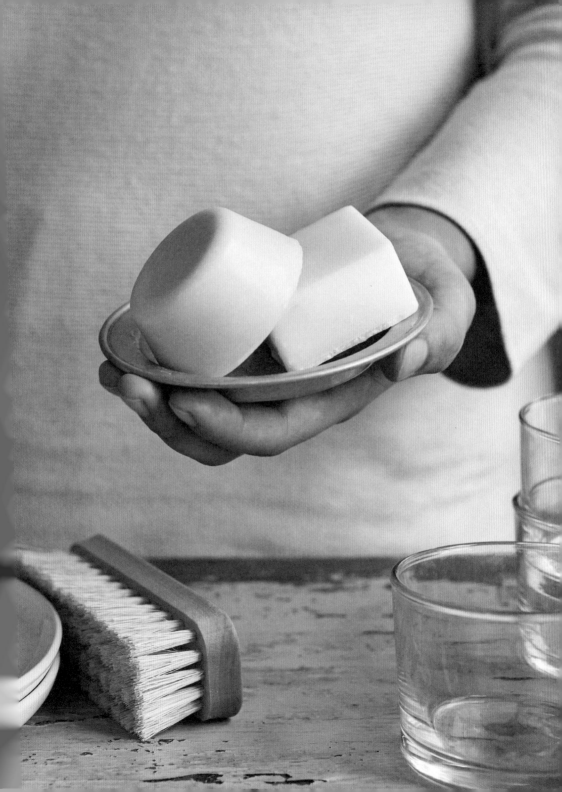

castile soap

Difficulty level: Beginner
Recipe makes: 200g (7.05oz) of soap,
1–3 soaps depending on the size of
the mould used
Cure time: 4–6 weeks
Shelf life: 6 months

ingredients
lye solution (40% concentration, 5% superfat)
- 38.61g (1.36oz) water
- 25.74g (0.91oz) sodium hydroxide

oils
- 100% olive oil: 200g (7.05oz)
- Optional: 6g (0.21oz) essential oils of your choice (3% of your total oil quantity, which in this case is 200g (7.05oz)
- Optional: 2.20g (0.07oz) sodium lactate, this will help increase the hardness of the soap

recommended soaping temperature
49°C (120°F)

equipment
- Goggles
- Gloves
- High precision scales
- 2 heat-safe glass or stainless steel jugs
- Ceramic or glass bowl
- Mask/respirator or scarf
- Stainless steel tablespoon
- Thermometer
- Stainless steel saucepan
- Silicone spatula
- Stick blender
- Moulds

tip
When choosing which olive oil to use, keep in mind that this soap will need to cure for four to six months or even up to one year, so it is important to use high quality, fresh olive oil. The best choice would be a pure olive oil from a reliable cosmetic supplier. If you are buying the olive oil from your local supermarket, avoid using lower quality olive oils packed in very large quantities because they often sit on the shelves for a very long time and might not be very fresh. You can use extra virgin olive oil or pomace oil; however, since these olive oil grades are unrefined, they might be more prone to spoilage.

This Castile soap recipe has a 40% water discount, so your lye solution will be much more concentrated and your soap will take less time to reach trace, harden up and cure.

The soap is also made at a higher temperature of 49°C (120°F), because a higher temperature will let the soap harden faster.

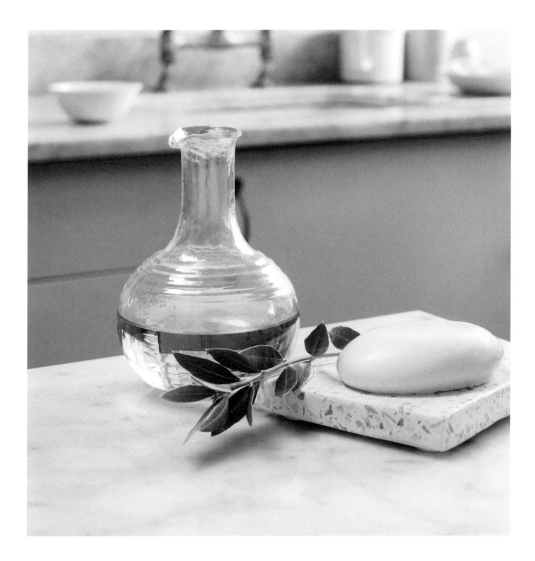

safety notes

Keep goggles and gloves on at all times when handling lye and raw soap.

Work in a well-ventilated area and keep children and pets away.

Do not weigh the sodium hydroxide in an aluminium container, or in a very light paper or plastic one.

Add the sodium hydroxide to the water and never the opposite.

This lye solution is more concentrated than normal and will therefore heat up faster. Please take extra care when preparing your lye solution.

instructions

1. Wearing goggles and gloves, weigh the sodium hydroxide (see Safety Notes, see pages 86–87).

2. Weigh the water in a separate heat-safe glass or stainless steel container.

3. Keep your gloves and goggles on, and wear your mask/respirator if you have one, or a scarf over your nose and mouth. To prepare the lye solution, add the sodium hydroxide to the water and stir with a stainless steel spoon until it is fully dissolved. Put the lye solution in a safe spot away from pets and children until it cools down to 49°C (120°F). Monitor the temperature using a thermometer.

4. When the lye solution has almost reached 49°C (120°F), weigh the olive oil in a clean stainless steel or heat-safe bowl and heat it up on the stove or in the microwave so it also reaches about 49°C (120°F). If you are using the microwave, heat it up in 20 second bursts so you can better control the temperature. If you want to add essential oils, weigh them at this point and keep them on the side ready to be used in one of the next steps. Prepare the moulds you want to use for your soaps.

5. Once the olive oil is around 49°C (120°F) add the lye solution to the olive oil and gently stir with a spatula.

6. Stick blend until you reach trace (see page 82) – as this is 100% olive oil soap, it might take longer than usual. If you want to add essential oils, add them at a very light trace and stick blend a little bit more. Stick blend until you reach a light-medium trace.

7. Pour the mixture into the moulds and tap to remove any air bubbles. Cover the soap with a piece of cardboard and add a blanket or a pile of fabric to keep the soap warm and insulated as much as possible. The heat will make the soap harden faster, which will also result in a faster cure time.

8. Unmould the soap after 48 hours. Although you can use Castile soap after 4-6 weeks, it can benefit from a longer cure time. This is due to the exclusive use of olive oil, which will take longer to properly harden up. I usually leave mine for at least 3 months, while some soap makers enjoy curing it even up to 6 months. The more humid your curing room is, the longer I would let the soap cure.

---

tip

I normally leave Castile soap unscented because essential oils will likely fade after such a long cure time.

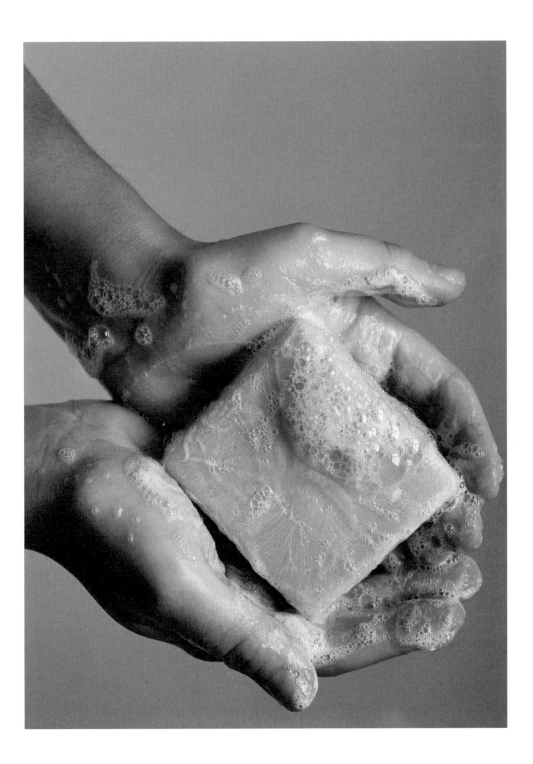

coconut body or dishwashing soap

Difficulty level: Beginner
Recipe makes: 200g (7.05oz) of soap,
approximately 4 soaps depending
on the size of the mould used
Cure time: 4–6 weeks
Shelf life: 6 months

ingredients
lye solution for a body soap (33% lye concentration, 20% superfat)
- 29.32g (1.03oz) sodium hydroxide
- 59.53g (2.10oz) water

lye solution for a dishwashing soap (33% lye concentration, 0% superfat)
- 36.65g (1.29oz) sodium hydroxide
- 74.41g (2.62oz) water

oil (this is the same for both recipes)
- 100% coconut oil: 200g (7.05oz)
- Optional: 6g (0.21oz) of essential oils (3% of your total oil quantity, which in this case is 200g/7.05oz)

recommended soaping temperature
- 38°C (100°F)

equipment
- Goggles
- Gloves
- High precision scales
- 2 heat-safe glass or stainless steel jugs
- Ceramic or glass bowl
- Mask/respirator or scarf
- Stainless steel tablespoon
- Thermometer
- Stainless steel saucepan
- Silicone spatula
- Stick blender
- Moulds

tip
You can use extra virgin coconut oil or a refined coconut oil. The only difference is that the extra virgin oil has not undergone a refinement process so will have a stronger scent, which means the coconut scent will likely mask any essential oil scent.

The body soap is superfatted at 20% (see page 83), which means it will not be drying at all and will be milder for the skin. On the contrary, the dish soap has a 0% superfat so it will be really cleansing.

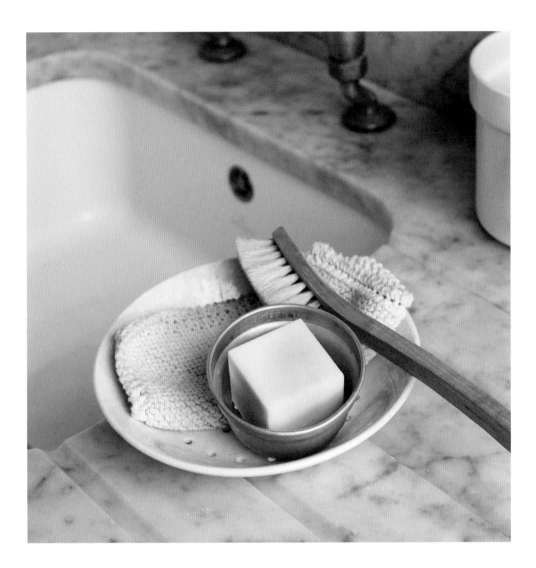

safety notes

For this recipe you can use up to 6g (0.21oz) of essential oils. Do not exceed this amount.

Keep goggles and gloves on at all times when handling lye and raw soap.

Work in a well-ventilated area and keep children and pets away.

Do not weigh the sodium hydroxide in an aluminium container, or in a very light paper or plastic one.

Add the sodium hydroxide to the water and never the opposite.

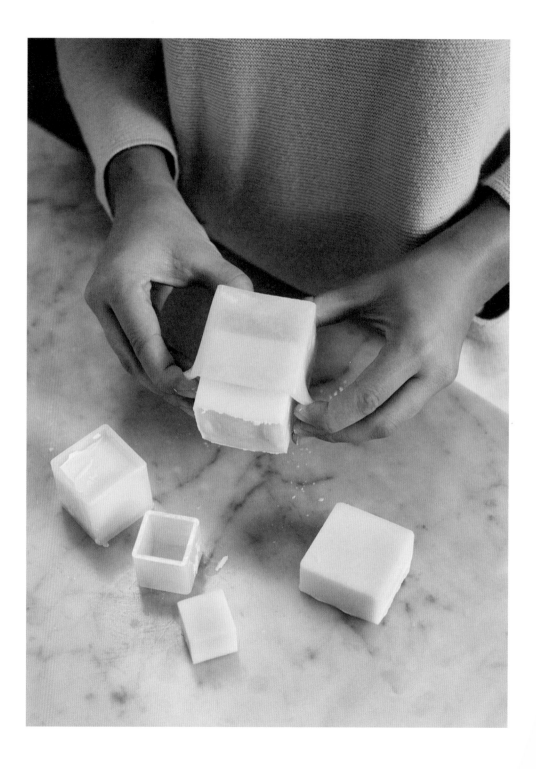

instructions

1. Wearing goggles and gloves, weigh the sodium hydroxide (see Safety Notes, pages 86–87).

2. Weigh the water in a separate heat-safe glass or stainless steel container.

3. Keep your gloves and goggles on, and wear your mask/respirator if you have one, or a scarf over your nose and mouth. To prepare the lye solution, add the sodium hydroxide to the water and stir well with a stainless steel tablespoon to dissolve it fully, make sure not to cause splashes. Put the lye solution in a safe spot away from pets and children until it cools down to 38°C (100°F). Monitor the temperature using a thermometer.

4. While the lye solution is cooling down, weigh the coconut oil in a clean stainless steel or heat-safe bowl and, if solid (it will be liquid during mild/hot temperatures), melt it slightly on the stove or in the microwave. I prefer to not melt it all the way through so that it does not overheat. This should take you a few seconds. At this point weigh your essential oils, if using, and keep them on the side ready to be used in one of the next steps. Prepare the moulds you want to use for your soaps.

5. Check that the coconut oil is at about 38°C (100°F), then add the lye solution to the coconut oil and gently stir with a spatula.

6. Stick blend until you reach trace (see page 82). If you want to add the essential oils, do this at a very light trace and stir them in with a spatula until fully incorporated. Stick blend for a few seconds making sure the soap retains a light trace and does not harden too much.

7. Pour the soap into the moulds and tap to remove any air bubbles. Leave the soap to air dry and do not cover it with anything – you want it to harden and not overheat, since the heat might crack it.

8. Unmould the soap after 24 hours, and then leave it to cure on a clean shelf in a dry room for 4–6 weeks.

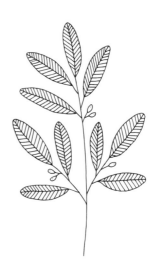

detoxifying soap

Difficulty level: Intermediate
Recipe makes: 250g (8.81oz) of soap,
about 4–6 soaps depending on the
size of the mould used
Cure time: 4–6 weeks
Shelf life: 6 months

You will soon realize the incredible therapeutic aspect of making soap – not only while you make it, but also when you use it. That's why making soaps to gift to family and friends is an incredibly rewarding experience both for the maker and the end user!

Although in soap making you can obtain natural colours using infusions, this method sometimes takes a lot of trial and error because many natural colours tend to fade with the soap-making reaction. In this project I show you how you can make a customizable soap using a clay or a powder of your choice. You will be able to choose between three combinations: pink clay, green clay or activated charcoal – these ingredients will all produce a wonderful soap with a detoxifying effect. I've kept the selection of the additive open to your choice, so you can truly customize the soap.

I kept the selection of oils in this recipe simple yet very nourishing. The combination of olive oil, coconut oil, shea butter and castor oil will produce a hard and bubbly bar of soap. As this is a coloured soap, I suggest soaping at slightly higher temperatures to encourage the soap to go through 'gel phase' (see page 85) and allow the colours to pop out more.

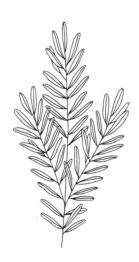

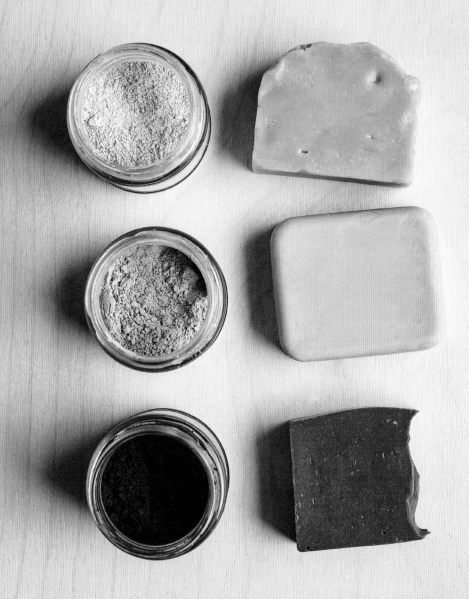

ingredients
lye solution (33% lye concentration, 5% superfat)

- 70.72g (2.49oz) water
- 34.83g (1.23oz) sodium hydroxide

oils

- 65% olive oil: 162.50g (5.73oz)
- 25% coconut oil: 62.50g (2.20oz)
- 5% shea butter: 12.50g (0.44oz)
- 5% castor oil: 12.50g (0.44oz)

additives, pick one of the following

- 3.44g (0.12oz) pink clay
- 5.36g (0.19oz) green clay
- 2.58g (0.09oz) activated charcoal
- Optional: 7.50g (0.26oz) of essential oils, see Suggested Essential Oil Blends, opposite (3% of your total oil quantity, which in this case is 250g/8.81oz)
- Optional: 2.76g (0.09oz) sodium lactate, to be added to the lye solution when cooled down (see step 3)

recommended soaping temperature

- 49°C (120°F)

safety notes

For this recipe you can use up to 6g (0.21oz) of essential oils. Do not exceed this amount.

Keep goggles and gloves on at all times when handling lye and raw soap.

Work in a well-ventilated area and keep children and pets away.

Do not weigh the sodium hydroxide in an aluminium container, or in a very light paper or plastic one.

Add the sodium hydroxide to the water and never the opposite.

equipment

- Gloves
- Goggles
- High precision scales
- 2 heat-safe glass or stainless steel jugs
- Ceramic or glass bowl
- Mask/respirator or scarf
- Stainless steel tablespoon
- Thermometer
- Stainless steel saucepan
- Silicone spatula
- Stick blender
- Moulds

suggested essential oil blends

Lavender and tea tree
Lavender and geranium
Eucalyptus, rosemary and peppermint
Lavender and rosemary

instructions

1. Wearing gloves and goggles, weigh the sodium hydroxide (see Safety Notes, pages 86–87).

2. Weigh the water in a separate heat-safe glass or stainless steel container. If you are using a clay to colour your soap, weigh your clay of choice in a small bowl and add it to the water. Mix well to dissolve it completely. If you choose to use charcoal, do not add it to the water; instead add it to your melted oils in step 4.

3. Keep your gloves and goggles on, and wear your mask/respirator if you have one, or a scarf over your nose and mouth. To prepare the lye solution, add the sodium hydroxide to the water and stir well with a stainless steel tablespoon to dissolve it fully, make sure not to cause splashes. Put the lye solution in a safe spot away from pets and children until it cools down to 49°C (120°F). Monitor the temperature using a thermometer.

4. While the lye solution is cooling down, weigh the oils in a clean stainless steel or heat-safe glass bowl, depending on how you would like to melt them (directly on the stove or in the microwave). If you are using activated charcoal, dissolve it into your oils once they are warm and completely melted.

5. If you are using essential oils, weigh them into a separate beaker/glass so you have them ready to pour into the soap when you reach a light trace. Prepare your moulds so you have them ready for later.

6. Check the temperature of the lye solution and the oils. They should be both at around 49°C (120°F). If adding sodium lactate, add this to the lye solution before pouring the lye onto the oils, making sure it is well mixed. Add the lye solution to the melted oils and gently stir with a spatula.

7. Stick blend until you reach a light trace (see page 82). Add the essential oils and mix with a spatula until fully incorporated. Stick blend a few more seconds until you reach a slightly thicker trace.

8. Pour the mixture into the moulds and tap to remove any air bubbles. As an optional step, you can spray the surface with 99.9% isopropyl alcohol to prevent any soda ash from forming – as these are coloured soaps soda ash would be very noticeable. Cover the soap with a piece of cardboard and add a blanket or a pile of fabrics to keep the soap warm and insulated as much as possible – this will also help to prevent any soda ash from forming.

9. Unmould the soap after 24 hours. At this point, leave it to cure on a clean shelf in a dry room for 4–6 weeks before trying it.

repurposed food waste soap

Difficulty level: Intermediate
Recipe makes: 300g (10.58oz) of soap,
  6–8 soaps depending on the size of
  the mould used
Cure time: 4–6 weeks
Shelf life: 6 months

When you start making soap you will soon realize
that what you can achieve in a simple bar of soap
is almost limitless. You can really easily create a
detoxifying charcoal soap for acne-prone skin or
even make soap out of food waste. In this project
we are going to explore how to make soap by
repurposing coffee grounds. If you are not a coffee
drinker, you can replace the coffee grounds with
ground tea leaves or any other ingredient with
exfoliating properties – I have included
some suggestions in the ingredients list.

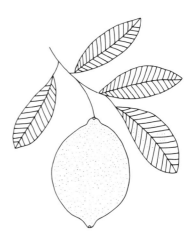

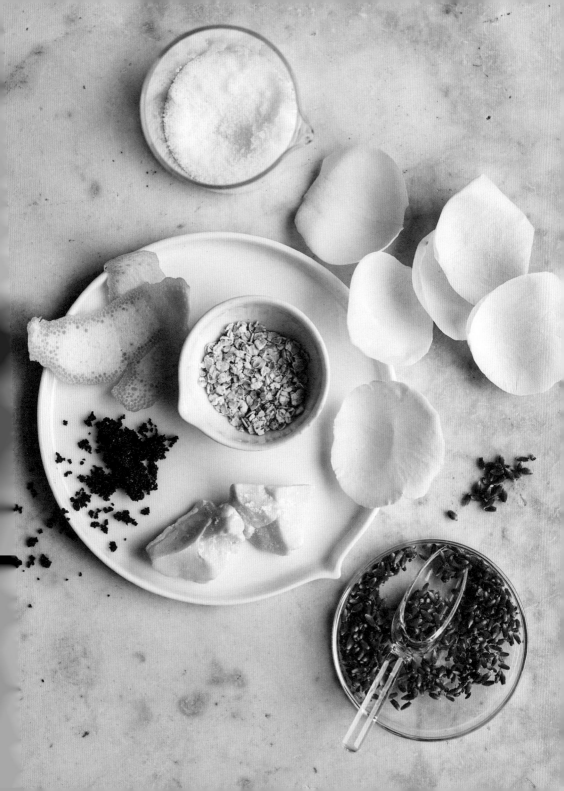

ingredients

lye solution (33% lye concentration, 5% superfat)

- 86.95g (3.07oz) water
- 42.83g (1.51oz) sodium hydroxide

oils

- 55% olive oil: 165g (5.82oz)
- 30% coconut oil: 90g (3.17oz)
- 10% cocoa butter: 30g (1oz)
- 5% sweet almond oil: 15g (0.53oz)

suggested essential oil blends

- Coffee soap: patchouli and bergamot
- Oatmeal soap: lavender and petitgrain
- Tea soap: grapefruitand geranium
- Lemon soap: lemongrass and lavender
- Orange soap: sweet orange and may chang

additives, pick one of the following

8g (0.28oz) of either:

- Dried coffee grounds
- Oatmeal pulp or ground oatmeal powder
- Finely ground tea leaves
- Desiccated lemon peel
- Orange zest
- Optional: 3.31g (0.116oz) sodium lactate, to be added to the lye solution when cooled down (see step 4)
- Optional: 9g (0.31oz) of essential oils, see Suggested Oil Blends, opposite (3% of your total oil quantity, which in this case is 300g/10.58oz)

recommended soaping temperature

- 43°C (110°F)

equipment

- Goggles
- Gloves
- High precision scales
- 2 heat-safe glass or stainless steel jugs
- Ceramic or glass bowl
- Mask/respirator or scarf
- Stainless steel tablespoon
- Thermometer
- Stainless steel saucepan
- Silicone spatula
- Stick blender
- Moulds

safety notes

For this recipe use up to 3g (0.10oz) of essential oils. Do not exceed this amount.

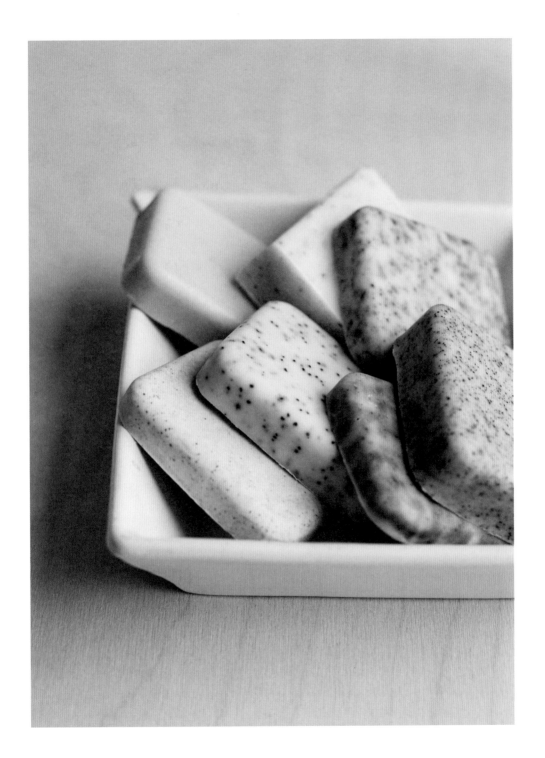

instructions

1. Wearing goggles and gloves, weigh the sodium hydroxide (see Safety Notes, pages 86–87).

2. Weigh the water in a separate heat-safe glass or stainless steel container.

3. Keep your gloves and goggles on, and wear your mask/respirator if you have one, or a scarf over your nose and mouth. To prepare the lye solution, add the sodium hydroxide to the water and stir well with a stainless steel tablespoon to dissolve it fully, make sure not to cause splashes. Put the lye solution in a safe spot away from pets and children.

4. Optional step: Weigh the sodium lactate in a small bowl/beaker. Once the lye solution has cooled down and before adding the oils, slowly mix in the sodium lactate and stir well.

5. While the lye solution is cooling down, weigh the oils in a clean stainless steel or heat-safe glass bowl, depending on how you would like to melt them. I normally melt the butters on the stove in a bain-marie (see page 29) along with the other oils.

6. While the butters/oils are melting, start preparing the additives. Weigh the food waste additive of your choice and keep it in a bowl. Weigh the essential oils of your choice – if you want you can add the essential oils to the bowl of food waste additives to avoid too much clutter. Finally, prepare the moulds for the soap.

7. Monitor the temperature of the lye solution and the oils using a thermometer. Once they are both at 43°C (110°F) (this will take roughly 20–30 minutes), add the lye solution onto the melted oils and gently stir with a spatula.

8. Stick blend until you reach a light trace (see page 82). Next, add your essential oils and food waste ingredients and mix with a spatula until fully incorporated. Stick blend a few more seconds until you reach a slightly thicker, yet still very pourable trace.

9. Pour the mixture into the moulds and tap to remove any air bubbles. Cover the soap with a piece of cardboard and add a blanket or a pile of fabrics to keep the soap warm and insulated as much as possible. This will also avoid any soda ash from forming (see page 87); on coloured soaps like this one it would ruin its appearance.

10. Unmould the soap after 24 hours. At this point, leave it to cure on a clean shelf in a dry room for 4–6 weeks before enjoying its invigorating exfoliating effect!

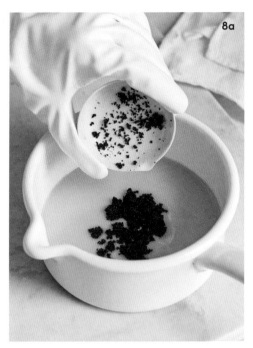

8a

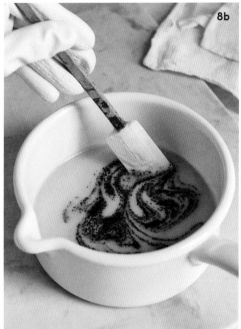

8b

tip

Whatever additive you decide to use, make sure that it is dry to avoid any mould forming in the final soap. If you are using a peel or zest, you can dry it in the oven and grind it into a fine powder once dry.

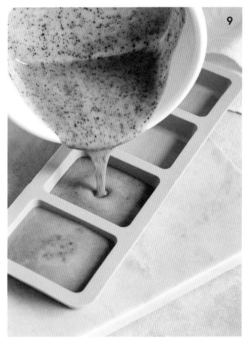

9

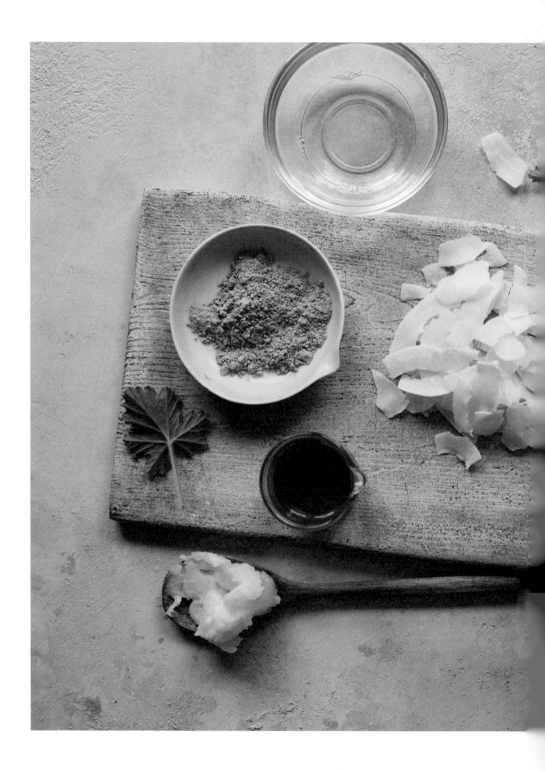

haircare

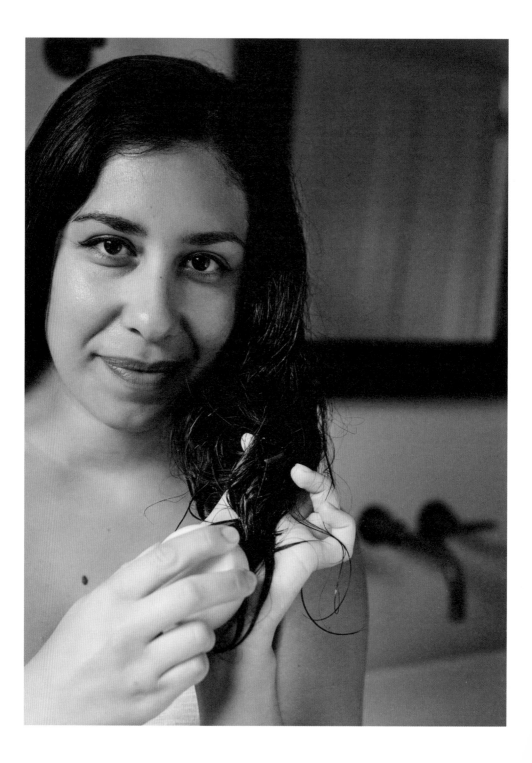

haircare

Haircare has always been a fascinating subject for me. I have long, thick, wavy hair, which has the tendency to become really frizzy with the slightest humidity. I dyed, coloured and styled my hair throughout my teenage years. Basically, I was never really fully satisfied with it, and always tried to make it into something it was not. When I started living zero waste I was faced with quite a big challenge: how will I take care of something that is already tricky for me to handle, while doing it in a natural and sustainable way?

shampoo

I first tried to make a shampoo bar out of soap. This is a very common approach in the zero-waste world, because it was adopted by many soap makers who were trying to expand their product lines to include shampoo bars. However, I quickly learned that soap making is definitely not the right method to make a shampoo bar. If you have already experimented with shampoo bars, you have probably found yourself running your fingers through sticky, tangled hair or have had a very dry scalp at least once.

There are two main things to consider when making a shampoo: the mildness and the pH. The pH is a figure expressing the acidity or alkalinity of a substance, which is calculated in a water-based solution. On a scale from 0 to 14, 7 is considered neutral. Vinegar, lemon or citric acid are acidic with a pH of 2, while something like sodium hydroxide has a basic/alkaline pH of 14. Skin is naturally acidic – it is often referred to as the acidic mantle – with a pH between 4 and 5.5. Hair likes acidic things, so any haircare product should have an acidic pH of 6 or lower. This is something impossible to achieve with soap bars, because natural cold process soap is made by mixing oils and sodium hydroxide. Oils do not have a pH but sodium hydroxide has a pH of 14, so the pH of a soap bar is around 8. Hair is made up of different layers (the medulla, the cortex and the cuticles), kind of like a rope, and a high pH will make the outer cuticle layer rise, too much water then gets inside the hair and it becomes swollen and damaged over time. So haircare products should really be crafted by selecting ingredients that already have an acidic pH of 6 or lower, or by adjusting the pH of the final product. Adjusting the pH of a final product can be a little tricky, so the projects in this section focus on crafting amazing haircare recipes using already pH-balanced ingredients.

In every good shampoo bar there should be three main components to:

1. Cleanse
2. Protect
3. Preserve

The cleanse part will be made up by detergents called surfactants. The main detergents used in these recipes are sodium cocoyl isethionate (SCI), an anionic (negatively charged) surfactant that is derived from coconut oil, and cocamidropopyl betaine, an amphoteric (with a variable charge) surfactant that is derived from coconut oil and fruit sugars. Both of these ingredients are pH balanced. The action of these surfactants is to clean the hair and the scalp, and blending them together will make this cleansing action milder.

In order to avoid the shampoo bar stripping the hair, a good, balanced shampoo bar should also have a mix of protective ingredients. These can be oils, proteins, vitamins, conditioning ingredients, to name just a few.

Finally, the formula includes a broad-spectrum preservative. In fact, any product that contains water or comes in contact with water should be correctly preserved to avoid any mould and bacteria growing. The preservative should be broad spectrum, because this means that it can protect against bacteria, yeast, fungus and mould. A non-broad spectrum preservative will protect you from some types of bacteria but could be, for example, weak against fungus. When incorporating preservatives it is important to pay attention to the recommended temperature: some will become inactive if added at too high a temperature. For this reason, the preservative will be the last ingredient added to your shampoo bars, normally when the mixture has cooled down below 45°C (113°F). Like many cosmetic ingredients, preservatives are often sold using trade names and this can be quite confusing. On the opposite page there are some eco-friendly preservatives you can use in your shampoo bars.

Finally, remember that vitamin E is not a preservative – it is an antioxidant and can be used to prevent oxidation and improve an oil's shelf life.

conditioner

Conditioners are truly an amazing way to keep your hair healthy in a low waste way: they are solid and concentrated and last for a very long time. In order to craft conditioner bars you will need to use positively charged/cationic ingredients. If you used a butter, such as cocoa butter or shea butter, or an oil, such as sweet almond oil, it would probably soften and nourish your hair but it would not really condition it. Chances are it will make your hair greasy or even a little crunchy, but a good conditioner will make your hair soft, frizz-free and very easy to brush through. Conditioner bars are made using fatty alcohols and conditioning ingredients, some of which harden at around 60°C (140°F) – so the preservative should be stable at this temperature or higher, otherwise you would not be able to let the bar cool down because it would become hard and unpourable. To correctly preserve your conditioner bars, choose a preservative from the list opposite.

preservatives

preservative name	INCI
Geogard 221 / Cosgard **(<)**	Dehydroacetic acid and Benzyl alcohol
Mikrokill ECT/ Geogard ECT/Plantaserv M **(<)***	Benzyl Alcohol (and) Salicylic Acid (and) Glycerin (and) Sorbic Acid
Liquid Germall ™Plus **(<)**	Propylene Glycol (and) Diazolidinyl Urea (and) Iodopropynyl Butylcarbamate
Phenonip ® **(<) (C)**	Phenoxyethanol (and) Methylparaben (and) Ethylparaben (and) Butylparaben (and) Propylparaben (and) Isobutylparaben
Naticide / Plantaserv Q **(<)**	Parfum
Optiphen™ **(<) (C)**	Phenoxyethanol (and) Caprylyl glycol
Optiphen™ Plus **(<) (C)**	Phenoxyethanol (and) Caprylyl glycol (and) Sorbic acid
Optiphen™ 300 **(<) (C)**	Phenoxyethanol and Caprylyl glycol
Euxyl PE9010 **(<) (C)**	Phenoxyethanol and Ethylhexylglycerin

Important: you are responsible for checking the efficacy of the preservative system you chose to use. Please ensure to check the correct usage rate with your supplier as this might vary, as well as the suitable pH range and temperature of inclusion. They will be able to provide you with all the information you need based on the product you are making.

Should you need to test the pH of your product, you can do so by creating a solution with 10% of your product and 90% distilled water (example: dissolve 1g/0.035oz of shampoo bar into 9g /0.31oz of distilled water) and then test the pH of the solution using pH strips, or better, with a pH meter. Should you need to adjust the pH,

then create a 50% distilled water to 50% citric acid solution, and add the solution into your final product (when still melted), 1 drop at a time, while testing the pH in a new 10% product to 90% distilled water solution, until you have reached the desired pH.

(<) To include only at temperatures below 45°C (104°F) or lower.

(C) Suitable to include at 60°C (140°F) in conditioner bars recipes.

* Not allowed in products for children under the age of three.

minimalist haircare routine

Before you dive into the first recipes, let's explore how you can take care of your hair and still maintain a minimalist and healthy haircare routine. You will soon realize you really don't need very many products at all – you could very easily use just three:

1. A shampoo bar
2. A conditioner bar
3. An oil

Here is something fascinating about hair and haircare products: to be really successful, they should complement each other. In chemistry, opposite charges attract each other, and like charges repel each other. Hair is negatively charged, just like the cleaning ingredients in shampoos – as a result, cleaning ingredients are able to repel the dirt off your hair. By contrast, conditioners are positively charged – so when they meet the negative charge of your hair the conditioning ingredients are attracted and will make the hair cuticle close and look healthier and shinier.

Finally, hair oils are great to keep your scalp moisturized and to soften dry ends. Virtually any oil can be used on hair, although – based on their fatty acid profile – some are considered more effective than others. For example, coconut oil is rich in lauric acid, which has an affinity for hair protein, and it has a low molecular weight so it is able to penetrate the hair shaft. Some other oils, such as avocado or olive oil, do not necessarily penetrate the hair shaft but are very moisturizing for the scalp because they are rich in oleic acid, which is incredibly emollient and can treat a dry, itchy, dandruff-prone, sensitivescalp. Jojoba, which is actually a liquid wax and not an oil, is amazing for haircare because it has a structure that is very similar to the skin's sebum, so it is said to be able to penetrate the hair follicles to provide hydration without clogging the pores. Broccoli seed oil is rich in erucic acid, which acts as a natural silicone to give amazing anti-frizz properties. Camellia seed oil has been used in Japan for centuries to tame frizzy hair and reduce dandruff, thanks to its high amounts of oleic acid. Castor oil is made up mostly of ricinoleic acid, which is said to thicken hair so is recommended if you are experiencing hair thinning.

dry ends
Coconut oil
Tomato seed oil
Argan oil
Camellia seed oil
Avocado oil
Broccoli seed oil
Grapeseed oil
Shea butter
Cocoa butter

dry, inflamed, itchy, dandruff scalp
Jojoba
Hemp seed oil
Sweet almond oil
Castor oil
Blackseed oil

hair growth/strengthening
Neem oil
Wheat germ oil
Castor oil
Blackseed oil
Flaxseed linseed oil